PRESIDENT'S MALARIA INITIATIVE

Zambia

Malaria Operational Plan FY 2015

TABLE OF CONTENTS

ACRONYMS

ACT	Artemisinin-based combination therapy
AIDS	Acquired Immuno-Deficiency Syndrome
AL	Artemether-lumefantrine
ANC	Antenatal care
BCC	Behavior change communication
CCT	Clinical care teams
CDC	U.S. Centers for Disease Control and Prevention
CHA	Community health assistant
CHAZ	Churches Health Association of Zambia
CHW	Community health worker
CSH	Communication Support for Health
DCMO	District Community Medical Offices
DDT	Dichloro-diphenyl-trichloroethane
DFID	U.K. Department for International Development
DHA-PQ	Dihydroartemisinin-piperaquine
DHIS2	Demographic and Health Information System 2
DHS	Demographic and Health Survey
DCHO	District Community Health Office
EMLIP	Essential Medicines Malaria Logistics Improvement Program
EPI	Expanded Program on Immunizations
EUV	End-use verification
FANC	Focused antenatal care
FBO	Faith-based organization
FETP	Field Epidemiology Training Program
FY	Fiscal year
GHI	Global Health Initiative
Global Fund	Global Fund to Fight AIDS, TB and Malaria
GRZ	Government of the Republic of Zambia
HIV	Human Immunodeficiency Virus
HMIS	Health Management Information System
iCCM	Integrated Community Case Management
IMaD	Improving Malaria Diagnostics Project
IMCI	Integrated management of childhood illnesses
IPTp	Intermittent preventive treatment for pregnant women
IRS	Indoor residual spraying
ITN	Insecticide-treated mosquito net
LLIN	Long-lasting insecticide-treated net
LMU	Logistics Management Unit
M&E	Monitoring and evaluation
MACEPA	Malaria Control and Evaluation Partnership in Africa
MCDMCH	Ministry of Community Development and Mother and Child Health
MIP	Malaria in pregnancy
MIS	Malaria Indicator Survey
MOH	Ministry of Health

MOP	Malaria operational plan
MSL	Medical Stores Limited
MTR	Mid-Term Review
NMCC	National Malaria Control Centre
NMCP	National Malaria Control Program
NMSP	National Malaria Strategic Plan
NGO	Non-governmental organization
OPD	Outpatient department
OR	Operational research
OTSS	Outreach training and supportive supervision
PEPFAR	President's Emergency Plan for AIDS Relief
PMI	President's Malaria Initiative
RA	Resident Advisor
RDT	Rapid diagnostic test
SMAG	Safe Motherhood Action Groups
SP	Sulfadoxine-pyrimethamine
TWG	Technical working group
UNICEF	United Nations Children's Fund
UNDP	United Nations Development Program
USAID	United States Agency for International Development
WHO	World Health Organization
WHOPES	World Health Organization Pesticide Evaluation Scheme
ZAC	Zambia Anglican Council
ZISSP	Zambia Integrated Systems Strengthening Project

EXECUTIVE SUMMARY

In May 2009, President Barack Obama announced the Global Health Initiative (GHI), a comprehensive effort to reduce the burden of disease and promote healthy communities and families around the world. Through the GHI, the United States Government will help partner countries improve health outcomes, with a particular focus on improving the health of women, newborns and children. The President's Malaria Initiative (PMI) is a core component of the GHI.

PMI was launched in June 2005 as a 5-year, $1.2 billion initiative to rapidly scale up malaria prevention and treatment interventions in high burden countries in sub-Saharan Africa. In December 2006, Zambia was selected as a PMI country. Since then, Zambia has received approximately $151 million in PMI funding.

Although there are signs of improvement, malaria continues to be a major cause of morbidity and mortality in Zambia and control of the disease remains one of the government's highest priorities. Overall, the number of reported malaria cases (clinical and confirmed) to the National Health Management Information System (HMIS) increased from 3,250,128 to 4,892,813 (2009-2013). The reported number of outpatient department (OPD) visits increased from 13,697,003 in 2009 to 21,668,763 in 2012. There have been substantial declines over the past three years of reported inpatient malaria deaths for all ages with a decrease from 3.9 per 10,000 to 2.8 per 10,000 (2010-2012). Malaria parasite prevalence by smear microscopy has declined from 22% to 15% during the years of 2006 – 2012, but has remained relatively unchanged during the period of 2010 – 2012 (16% - 15%) according to the 2012 Malaria Indicator Survey (MIS). Severe anemia also for children under the age of five years declined from 14% to 7% during the years of 2006 to 2012. The most up-to-date information on nationwide coverage of malaria prevention and control measures in Zambia comes from the 2012 MIS, which shows improvements. More than 68% of households own at least one insecticide-treated net (ITN) compared to 64% in 2010; 57% of children under five years of age slept under an ITN the night before the survey in 2012, compared to 50% in 2010. In 2012, almost 74% of households owned at least one ITN or were sprayed with an insecticide in the previous 12 months. Seventy-two percent of pregnant women took two or more doses of intermittent preventive treatment for pregnant women (IPTp).

The Fiscal Year (FY) 2015 PMI funding for Zambia complements the National Malaria Strategic Program for 2011-2016. The plan is also based on PMI experiences in its first five years. A planning visit took place in June 2014 with representatives from USAID and the Centers for Disease Control and Prevention (CDC), who met with the National Malaria Control Program (NMCP) (including the Ministry of Health (MOH) and the Ministry of Community Development, Mother and Child Health (MCDMCH)), and a variety of other partners involved in malaria prevention and control in the country. This is the eighth Malaria Operational Plan (MOP) for Zambia and describes proposed expenditures of $24 million for FY 2015 under PMI.

Insecticide-treated nets: In 2014, the NMCP and partners will distribute over 7 million insecticide treated nets (ITNs) through mass distribution campaigns and routine distribution at antenatal care (ANC) and Expanded Program of Immunization (EPI) clinics. PMI is contributing approximately 1.6 million with an additional 600,000 from the President's Emergency Plan for

AIDS Relief (PEPFAR). The mass campaign will occur in eight of the ten provinces as two provinces were completed in 2013. PMI supported the development of the Zambia Continuous/Routine Distribution Guideline that adds school and community distribution channels to ANC/EPI. With FY 2015 funding, PMI will provide technical assistance for the roll out of primary school and community distribution, as well as strategies for care and maintenance of nets. In addition, PMI will continue to monitor the durability of ITNs distributed during the mass campaign.

Indoor residual spraying: Over the last year, PMI supported the NMCP Indoor Residual Spraying (IRS) operations in 20 PMI focus districts (seven in Eastern Province; five in Muchinga Province; eight in Northern Province). Approximately   structures were sprayed, out of the targeted 529,564 (81.7% coverage) protecting 1,842,821 people (approximately 10% of the Zambian population). In January 2014 PMI expanded its support to an additional nine districts in two provinces with DFID funding, bringing the total to 29 districts (total of 40 districts following the Government of Zambia's recent district re-demarcation exercise). The MOH committed significant funding to IRS in 2014. With funding from the Zambian government, the NMCP initiated the procurement of $10 million worth of organophosphates for use in the 2014 spray season in non-PMI supported areas. With FY2015 funding, PMI will cover the cost of IRS in the 20 old boundary districts in five provinces: Central (2 districts), Eastern, Luapula, Muchinga and Northern. Approximately 450,000 structures will be targeted protecting more than two million people.

Malaria in Pregnancy: The NMCP has updated their recommendations for IPTp to recommend sulfadoxine-pyrimethamine (SP) at the 16th week of gestation, with subsequent monthly doses given up to the time of delivery, in accordance with recent changes in the World Health Organization (WHO) recommendations. The 73% national coverage of two doses of IPTp hides substantially lower rates in rural areas and among poorer women. Two major barriers to increasing three-dose IPTp coverage are late attendance of women for ANC and stockouts of SP. In 2014, PMI supported training of provincial- and district-level clinical care teams in providing supervision for IPTp, training of healthcare workers in IPTp, and behavior change and communication (BCC) activities to encourage early and frequent ANC attendance to receive IPTp. With FY 2015 funding, PMI will support supervision and training of health workers in the new NMCP guidelines for IPTp and BCC activities related to malaria in pregnancy.

Case management – Diagnostics: NMCP Guidelines for the Diagnosis and Treatment of Malaria in Zambia recommend parasitological diagnosis for all suspected malaria cases where confirmatory capacity is available. Diagnostic availability has increased over the past year with the procurement of nearly 11 million RDTs in 2013. The Government of the Republic of Zambia (GRZ) procured RDTs, and in addition PMI supported procurement and distribution of 3.5 million RDTs. PMI also supported the training of clinical and laboratory personnel in the use of diagnostic tools, and training of national, provincial, and district level staff in providing outreach training and support supervision (OTSS) for quality assurance of malaria diagnostics. With FY 2015 funding, PMI will procure about 3.5 million RDTs and reagents and supplies for microscopy. PMI will continue to strengthen OTSS of health workers, together with quality control of laboratory diagnosis.

Case management – Treatment: In 2014, the NMCP and partners made revisions to the Guidelines for the Diagnosis and Treatment of Malaria in Zambia that included: injectable artesunate for severe malaria, dihydroartemisinin-piperaquine (DHA-PQ) as an alternate first-line treatment of uncomplicated malaria, and rectal artesunate for pre-referral treatment of severe malaria. PMI procured 4,425,570 artemisinin-based combination therapies (ACTs) in 2014 for the treatment of malaria in health facilities and in the community. In addition, 4.3 million ACTs were procured with DFID funding, GRZ was planning to procure over 9 million, and Malaria No More (MNM) purchased 1.6 million. If all procurements arrive in country as planned, Zambia will have full supply of ACTs for the first time. With FY 2015 funding, PMI will purchase 2.5 million ACT treatments and 120,000 60mg vials of injectable artesunate. The priority going forward for PMI will be improving diagnostics, supportive supervision, roll out of injectable artesunate, and expanding access to treatment through integrated community case management (iCCM).

Case management – Pharmaceutical Management: In 2014 PMI provided support to the MOH, Medical Stores Limited (MSL) and other stakeholders to improve the collection, management and use of logistics data through the development of an electronic Logistics Management Information System (eLMIS). In 2014, MOH with support from partners redesigned the essential medicines malaria logistics improvement program (EMLIP), now referred to as the EMLIP hybrid. The MOH officially adopted the hybrid system and allowed the rollout of the EMLIP hybrid system to resume. The Logistcs Management Unit at the MOH recorded 98% reporting rate and improved commodity facility level stock availability (97%) for EMLIP districts for the period January to June of 2014. PMI continued to provide technical assistance at the national level through participation in working groups related to procurement and supply chain management. With FY2015 funding, PMI will continue to support strengthening the GRZ's commodities supply and logistics systems at central, provincial, district and health center level.

Behavior Change Communication: The NMCP has a well-defined and thoughtful BCC strategy. It addresses the challenges Zambia currently faces and clearly anticipates those it will face as Zambia moves forward in malaria control. Recent evidence from the MIS 2012 shows that knowledge among women 15 – 49 years of age of malaria preventive and curative actions has been maintained at a high level. In FY 2015, PMI will continue to support NMCP's BCC strategy through integrated activities at national, community and individual levels for each malaria control intervention. PMI will support programs to increase use of ANC services including IPTp, to encourage constant and continuous use of long-lasting insecticide-treated nets (LLINs) every night year-round and to inform caregivers of the importance of seeking care quickly for children with fever.

Monitoring & Evaluation: Zambia has strong monitoring and evaluation (M&E) activities. A Mid-Term Review (MTR) of the National Malaria Strategic Plan (NMSP) 2011-2015 was completed in October 2013. A demographic health survey (DHS) that includes a malaria module is on-going in 2014. Zambia's fifth MIS is planned for 2015. The national HMIS has been upgraded from the District Health Information System (DHIS) 1.4 to 2.0, offering significant improvements in timeliness of reporting, data visualization and data systems management. With FY 2015 funding, PMI will provide support to strengthen routine malaria data collection at the health facility, district, and provincial levels through the HMIS, support a health facility survey in 2016, monitor physical integrity of ITNs following the mass campaign, and support the training of two NMCP staff through the Zambia Field Epidemiology Training Program (FETP).

STRATEGY

1. Introduction

Zambia was selected as a President's Malaria Initiative (PMI) country in fiscal year (FY) 2007. PMI in Zambia has supported the scale up of all major malaria prevention, control, diagnosis, and treatment modalities.

This fiscal year (FY) 2015 Malaria Operational Plan (MOP) presents a detailed implementation plan for Zambia, based on the PMI Multi-Year Strategy and Plan and the National Malaria Control Program's (NMCP's) 2011–2016 National Malaria Strategic Plan (NMSP). The MOP was developed in consultation with the NMCP, with participation of national and international partners involved in malaria prevention and control in the country. The proposed activities build on investments made by PMI and other partners to improve and expand malaria-related services, including the Global Fund to Fight AIDS, Tuberculosis, and Malaria (Global Fund) and focused support by the United Kingdom's Department for International Development (DFID). This document reviews the current status of malaria control policies and interventions in Zambia, describes progress to date, identifies challenges and unmet needs if the targets of the NMCP and PMI are to be achieved, and provides a description of planned FY 2015 activities.

2. Country Development Indicators and Malaria Situation

Zambia has a 2014 estimated population of 14.6 million (2010 census with 2.8% growth), with 40% residing in urban and 60% in rural areas. The country consists of ten provinces and 106 districts (recent redistricting has increased the number of districts from 72 original districts). Recently, Zambia has made progress towards the Millennium Development Goals (MDG) targets for 2015. According to UNICEF, under-five mortality has fallen from 192 deaths per 1,000 live births in 1992 to 89 deaths per 1,000 live births in 2012 (UNICEF, United Nations Population Division and United Nations Statistics Division). Eighty-six percent of children complete primary school (2007 Demographic and Health Survey - DHS). Lastly, Zambia has exceeded the MDG target for HIV/AIDS prevalence of 15.6% with an estimated 14.3% of the population living with HIV/AIDS. Despite these positive trends, Zambia continues to face major challenges. There continues to be an economic divide between the urban and rural populations, with the proportion of population living in extreme poverty at 13.1% for urban and 57.7% for rural areas (MDG Progress Report, Zambia, 2013).

Malaria transmission in Zambia occurs throughout the year with the peak during the rainy season, between November and April. The disease remains endemic but with wide variation in prevalence of infection across districts (Malaria Indicator Survey - MIS 2012). In Zambia, malaria is caused by the four main *Plasmodium* species that infect humans, with *Plasmodium falciparum* accounting for 98% of all infections. *Anopheles gambiae* and *An. funestus* are the major vectors. All ten provinces of Zambia are endemic for malaria with 90% of the population at risk. The NMCP first classified the country into three malaria epidemiological zones to better focus their efforts after the 2010 MIS. This classification has been updated following the 2012 MIS with North-Western Province dropping from Zone 2 to Zone 3.

- Zone 1: Areas where malaria control has markedly reduced transmission, and parasite prevalence in children less than five years of age is less than 1% (Lusaka city and environs).
- Zone 2: Areas where sustained malaria prevention and control has markedly reduced transmission, and parasite prevalence is at or under 14% in children under five years of age at the peak of transmission (Central, Copperbelt, Southern, and Western Provinces).
- Zone 3: Areas where progress in malaria control has been achieved but not sustained and lapses in prevention coverage have led to resurgence of infection and illness, and parasite prevalence in young children exceeds 14% at the peak of the transmission season (Eastern, Luapula, Muchinga, Northern, and North-Western Provinces).

Figure 1: National Malaria Control Program country classification of malaria epidemiological zones, 2013.

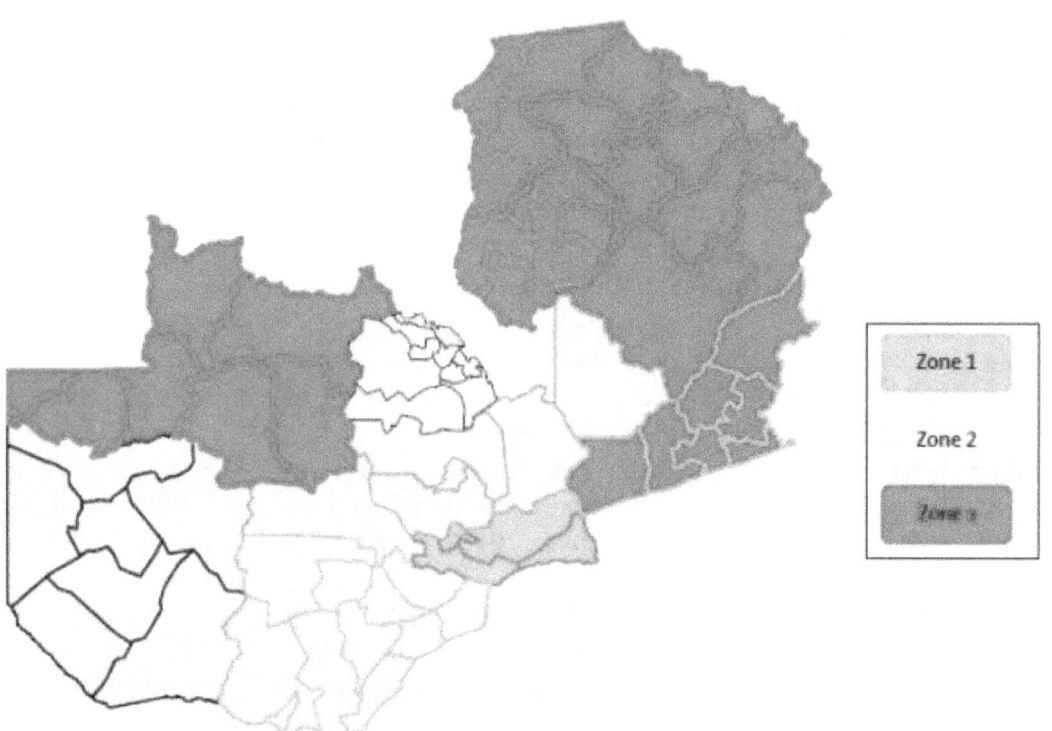

Overall, the number of reported malaria cases (clinical and confirmed) to the National Health Management Information System (HMIS) increased from 3,250,128 to 4,892,813 (2009-2013). The reported number of outpatient department (OPD) visits increased from 13,697,003 in 2009 to 21,668,763 in 2012. There have been substantial declines over the past three years of reported inpatient malaria deaths for all ages with a decrease from 3.9 per 10,000 to 2.8 per 10,000 (2010-2012). Malaria parasite prevalence by smear microscopy has declined from 22% to 15% during the years of 2006 – 2012, but has remained relatively unchanged during the period of 2010 – 2012 (16% - 15%) according to the 2012 MIS. Severe anemia for children under the age of five years also declined from 14% to 7% during the years of 2006 to 2012. This was especially notable in the provinces that reported higher insecticide-treated net (ITN) coverage compared to 2010, and in particular in the higher prevalence area of Luapula Province. It is important to note that these national-level numbers are not representative of all the trends across the country and there are documented variations between provinces and districts. For instance, the largest relative decline in parasite prevalence by microscopy was observed in Luapula Province (51% - 32%) compared to 2010. North-Western Province had the largest relative increase in parasite prevalence (6% - 17%), while Northern Province remained relatively unchanged (24%).

Background characteristic	Percentage with malaria parasites read by microscopy	Percentage with malaria parasites read by microscopy	Percentage with malaria parasites read by microscopy (or RDT)	Percentage with malaria parasites read by microscopy (or RDT)
	2006	2008	2010	2012
Age (in months)				
<12	12.6	3.6	5.7 (12.5)	9.8 (15.9)
12–23	22.8	10.2	12.1 (21.9)	11.7 (24.4)
24–35	25.3	11.2	20.1 (30.8)	16.3 (31.7)
36–47	26.3	13.8	21.4 (36.1)	16.2 (35.0)
48–59	24.4	12.5	22.0 (33.7)	19.6 (38.0)
Sex				
Male	21.9	10.5	16.9 (26.8)	14.7 (29.1)
Female	21.8	9.8	15.1 (26.7)	15.1 (30.0)
Residence				
Urban	6.4	4.3	5.2 (12.0)	3.7 (8.2)
Rural	27.8	12.4	20.4 (32.7)	20.2 (39.7)
Province				
Central	27.7	7.9	9.4 (11.5)	8.5 (12.8)
Copperbelt	12.4	9.9	12.1 (24.0)	4.7 (17.4)
Eastern	21.0	9.3	22.0 (50.1)	25.3 (51.1)
Luapula	32.9	21.8	50.5 (63.4)	32.1 (56.0)
Lusaka	0.8	1.7	0.0 (1.4)	0.0 (4.8)
Muchinga				19.4 (33.5)
Northern	35.3	12.0	23.6 (32.6)	23.7 (47.3)
North-Western	24.3	15.2	6.1 (17.3)	16.9 (32.5)
Southern	13.7	7.9	5.7 (12.2)	8.4 (10.0)
Western	11.1	2.6	5.1 (11.8)	12.6 (34.3)
Wealth index				
Lowest	30.4	13.1	29.2 (42.1)	27.4 (49.5)
Second	27.6	13.6	21.8 (36.2)	21.1 (42.8)
Middle	23.4	12.1	12.1 (22.9)	17.9 (35.1)

Table A: Malaria parasite prevalence in children under five years of age by background characteristic. Rapid Diagnostic Test (RDT) results in parenthesis, 2006 – 2012.

Table A: Malaria parasite prevalence in children under five years of age by background characteristic. Rapid Diagnostic Test (RDT) results in parenthesis, 2006 – 2012.				
Background characteristic	Percentage with malaria parasites read by microscopy	Percentage with malaria parasites read by microscopy	Percentage with malaria parasites read by microscopy (or RDT)	Percentage with malaria parasites read by microscopy (or RDT)
	2006	2008	2010	2012
Fourth	7.5	6.7	9.4 (20.6)	13.9 (27.7)
Highest	6.2	2.8	1.4 (4.4	1.8 (5.8)
Total	22.1	10.2	16.0 (26.7)	14.9 (29.5)

In addition, there has been an increase in the number of reported confirmed and clinical cases and deaths in North-Western Province. The HMIS also shows a trend in this geographic area of increasing malaria incidence during the period of 2011 – 2013. There has been an uptick in the number of reported clinical cases and deaths in Central Province over the past two years and should be monitored to ensure that there is not a reversal of the progress that has been made in this area during the preceding years. Reported malaria inpatients and deaths have declined over the past 5 years and this could be due in part to improved case management at the health facility level. The following table shows HMIS reporting of cases (clinical and confirmed), inpatients, and deaths during the period of 2009 – 2013.

Table B: Health Management Information Systems (HMIS) reported cases, deaths and inpatients, 2006 – 2012. Reporting rate as of 2013 at 90% (World Health Organization)					
Period	2009	2010	2011	2012	2013
Cases (clinical and confirmed)					
HMIS malaria cases total clinical	2,256,798	2,967,065	2,207,992	2,063,921	2,345,972
HMIS malaria cases total confirmed	993,330	1,330,092	2,227,904	2,696,983	2,546,841
HMIS malaria cases total	3,250,128	4,297,157	4,435,896	4,760,904	4,892,813
Inpatient cases and deaths					
HMIS malaria inpatient cases total	171,242	185,488	174,040	158,001	135,814
HMIS malaria deaths	5,088	5,133	4,357	3,898	3,242
Inpatient cases and deaths (<5yr)					
HMIS malaria inpatient cases total, <5yr	98,827	107,068	99,067	86,385	74,084
HMIS malaria deaths, <5yrs	2,847	2,949	2,580	2,248	2,032

Figure 2: Health Management Information System (HMIS) reported malaria incidence (per 1,000) by district during 2013.

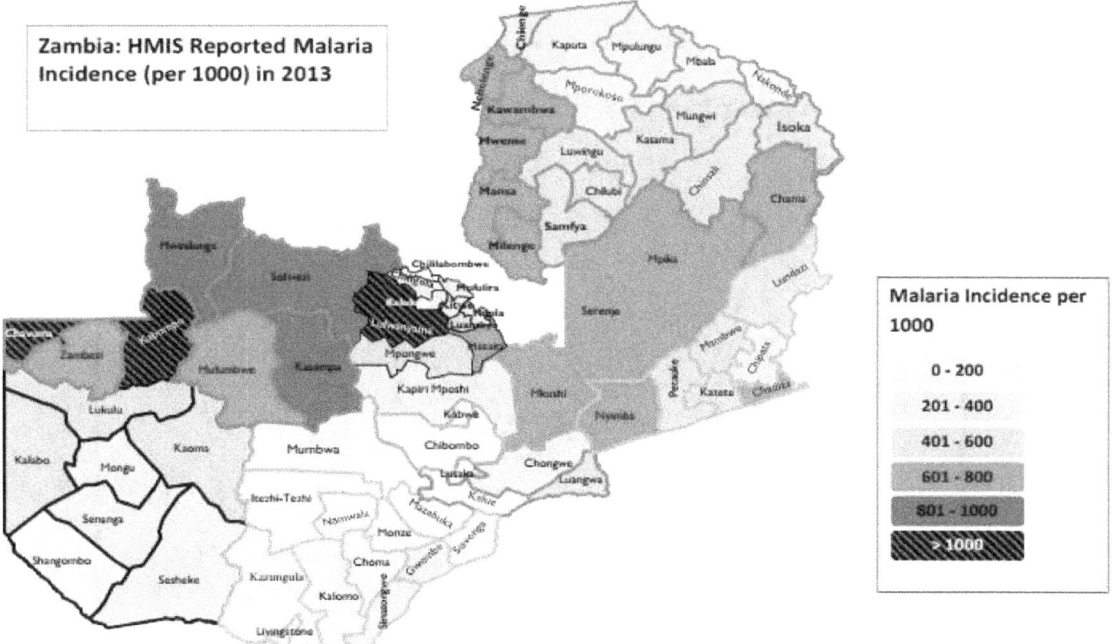

3. Country Health System Delivery Structure and Organization

Following the change of government in October 2011, the Zambian Government re-aligned the health portfolio functions between the Ministry of Health (MOH) and the Ministry of Community Development Mother and Child Health (MCDMCH). Under the new arrangement, the Ministry of Health is responsible for planning, health policy guidelines, surveillance, monitoring and evaluation, allocating funds, and sourcing key health inputs including drugs and equipment for service delivery. The MCDMCH is responsible for providing technical oversight for the implementation of health activities at district, health center, health post, and community levels.

Figure 3: Health Structure and Organization

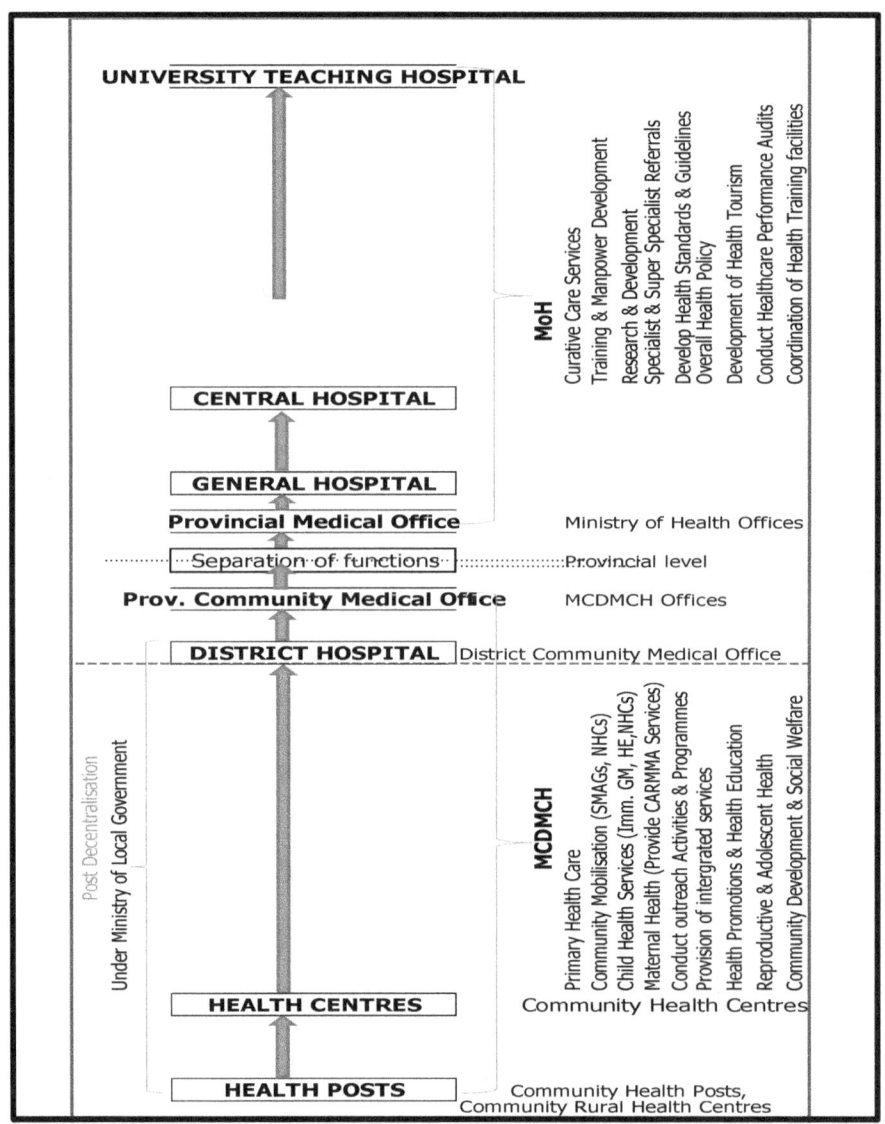

Government-run health facilities, which provide the majority of the health care in Zambia, offer a basic health care package of high-impact interventions. Services included in this basic health care package are provided free-of-charge or on a cost-sharing basis depending on the location and level of the system. In rural districts these services are free. The following are the levels of health care facilities offered throughout the country. Malaria control interventions are delivered in all of them.

- Community
- Health posts (district level)
- Health centers (district level)
- Level 1 hospitals (district level), Level 2 hospitals (provincial level), and Level 3 hospitals (central level)

Activities such as implementation of IRS, ITN distribution and malaria case management at level 1 hospitals, health centers, and community levels will now be the responsibility of MCDMCH implemented through the District Community Medical Offices (DCMOs). The MOH/National Malaria Control Centre (NMCC) will provide technical but not operational assistance at these levels.

Provincial Health Offices serve as an extension of the MOH. DCMOs are commissioned by the MCDMCH to provide services at the district and community level. The second- and third-level hospitals are referral or specialized hospitals. Due to resource constraints, however, there is generally a variation between what the levels are supposed to provide and what they actually do provide. Table B shows the breakdown by type of facility and provider.

Table C: Summary of health facilities by type and provider, Zambia, 2012		
Facility Type	Total	Percentage of Facilities
Health Posts	307	16
Rural Health Centers	1,131	58
Urban Health Centers	409	21
Level 1 Hospitals	84	4
Level 2 Hospitals	19	<1
Level 3 Hospitals	6	<1
Total	1,956	100
Health Facilities By Provider		
MOH	1,956	81
Mission	116	6
Private	250	13
Total	1,956	100

Source: Ministry of Health, 2012

The DCMO provides overall planning, coordination, and monitoring of malaria activities within their districts. Health posts are intended to cover 500–1,000 households. A newly created cadre of Community Health Assistants (CHAs) trained for one year and on government pay role has been deployed at some Health Posts in selected districts. At community level, community health workers (CHWs) provide malaria diagnostic and treatment services through the Integrated Community Case Management (ICCM) program. Health centers, staffed by a clinical officer, nurse, or environmental health technician, serve a catchment area of 10,000 residents. In 2010, it was estimated that in urban areas, approximately 99% of households are within five kilometers of a health facility, compared to 50% in rural areas. In 2012, Lusaka Province had the highest number of health facilities (294) followed by Southern (253), and the Copperbelt Province (250). Muchinga, the newly created province, had the lowest number of health facilities (99).

In addition to the MOH, the Churches Health Association of Zambia (CHAZ), parastatal organizations, private clinics, and traditional healers also provide health care in Zambia. CHAZ is an inter-denominational umbrella organization for coordinating church health services in Zambia that has 144 health facilities including hospitals, health centers, health posts and community-based organizations, and 11 health training schools, most of which are staffed by Government of Zambia health workers. Altogether, these institutions are responsible for over 50% of formal health services in the rural areas of Zambia and about 30% of health care in the country as a whole.

There over 600 for-profit private health facilities in Zambia, most of which are clinics attending to outpatients only, and located mainly in the urban districts. In addition, private mining companies provide preventive and curative medical services for their workers and families, as well as surrounding communities in some cases. Several of the larger mining companies, such as Konkola and Mopane Copper Mines, have been carrying out indoor residual spraying (IRS) for many years within and around their compounds.

4.   Country Malaria Control Strategy

The 2011-2015 National Malaria Strategic Plan (NMSP) underwent a midterm review in 2013. As a result of the review, the NMSP was extended by an additional year to run through 2016. The vision of the revised NMSP is to achieve progress towards a "malaria-free Zambia" through equity of access to quality-assured, cost-effective malaria prevention and control interventions close to the household. The NMSP aims to achieve the following three goals by 2016: 1) reduce malaria incidence by 75% from the 2010 baseline; 2) reduce malaria deaths to near zero and reduce all-cause child mortality by 20%; and 3) establish and maintain five "malaria-free zones" in Zambia.

The following overall changes were made to the NMSP following the 2013 mid-term review:
* A clear statement that the MCDMCH is now part of the NMCP,
* Emphasis on achieving and maintaining universal ITN coverage while utilizing a focal data driven approach to prioritize IRS,
* Greater attention paid to the coordination, leadership, governance and resource mobilization role of the NMCP for effective and efficient management, and
* Emphasis on ICCM rather than community management of malaria.

The NMCP aims to strengthen national-, provincial-, and district-level capacity to plan, manage, and implement malaria activities; address human resource needs; ensure that there is an established planning and forecasting framework for projecting funding needs and tracking health expenditures; develop capacity at all levels of the health system to manage the storage and distribution of malaria commodities; and reinforce coordination among partners. The plan seeks to have 100% of households and persons at risk in targeted areas have access to evidence-based vector control and other preventive interventions by 2016. The NMCP will aim to achieve and sustain universal ITN coverage and utilize a focal data-driven approach to prioritize IRS. The plan also seeks to improve malaria case management, diagnostic testing capacity and quality as well as increase coverage of three doses of sulfadoxine-pyrimethamine (SP) for intermittent preventive treatment in pregnancy (IPTp). In addition, the plan notes the need to strengthen behavior change communication (BCC) for malaria prevention and treatment, and the importance of establishing a robust surveillance, and monitoring and evaluation framework.

5.   Integration, Collaboration, Coordination

The NMCP and its collaborating partners maintain regular communications and coordinate efforts through routine partners' meetings and technical working groups (TWGs) on IRS, BCC, M&E, case management, ITNs, and operations research. The TWGs serve as technical advisory groups for the NMCP, ensuring implementation of quality malaria intervention. PMI and PMI-supported implementing partners play an important role in discussions and decision-making in the TWGs. For example, all partners including PMI, contributed to the development and mid-term review of the current 2011 – 2016 NMSP and annual action plans.

In 2014, PMI met regularly with World Health Organization (WHO), United Nations Development Program (UNDP), MOH, MCDMCH, and the Malaria Control and Evaluation Partnership in Africa (MACEPA) staff to assist with completion of the 2015 malaria Global Fund application. In addition, PMI regularly meets with these and other stakeholders such as the Clinton Health Access Initiative, World Vision and CHAZ to ensure coordination of malaria activities, including IRS and supply chain strengthening.

PMI met with the leaders of the Isdell-Flowers Cross Border Initiative, Christian Aid, and ExxonMobil to develop partnerships encourage ongoing collaboration with private sector donors in April 2012. PMI, through its implementing partners, has since continued and expanded this effort to include industry. Further, collaboration with the Clinton Health Access Initiative has resulted in an increased focus on sustainable financing and social responsibility. PMI is also working closely with the President's Emergency Plan for AIDS Relief (PEPFAR) to purchase and distribute PEPFAR-funded ITNs and to support focused antenatal care (FANC) strengthening efforts, since both programs utilize this platform in service delivery.

The Government of Zambia plans to provide annual funding dedicated to the procurement of key malaria control commodities (artemisinin-based combination therapies - ACTs, rapid diagnostic tests - RDTs, long-lasting insecticide-treated nets - LLINs, and IRS), and operational costs, increasing the investment it has made the past two fiscal years ($24 million – 2013, $27 million – 2014, and is planning for $28 million in 2015, $28.5 million in 2016, and $29 million in 2017). Zambia has a Transitional Funding Mechanism and is in the process of applying for a Global Fund Concept Note for the period of 2015 – 2017. The amounts requested are as follows in Table D below. These amounts are subject to change and are in the process of being negotiated between Zambia and the Global Fund.

Other major donors include DFID, the Bill and Melinda Gates Foundation through MACEPA, the World Health Organization (WHO), UNICEF, and private sector donations which are predominantly comprised of mining companies. DFID channels most of its malaria resources through PMI, thereby enhancing both agencies' buying power and making coordination of procurements much simpler and transparent. This tactical alliance will continue under this MOP, but is uncertain in future years due to changing funding portfolio at DFID. Table E depicts the anticipated level of funding for the years 2015 – 2017 from the various partners of NMCP.

Table D: Funding requested by the Government of Zambia to the Global Fund in support of malaria elimination activities			
Activity Area	Allocation	Above Allocation	Full Request
Vector Control	17,477,308	88,501,166	105,978,474
Case Management	19,200,743	41,457,947	60,658,690
Community Systems Strengthening	4,550,000	10,150,000	14,700,000
Health Systems Strengthening		5,500,000	5,500,000
Program Management	4,736,074		4,736,074
Monitoring and Evaluation	5,526,055		5,526,055
Total Funding	**51,490,180**	**145,609,113**	**197,099,293**

Note: the current Global Fund Allocation the current funding available support of malaria interventions, while the Above Allocation is the estimated amount that is required to implement the plan for consideration described in the Global Fund Concept Note.

Table E: Total Estimated Available Funding for Malaria Activities				
Partner	2015	2016	2017	Total
GRZ	28,000,000	28,500,000	29,000,000	85,500,000
PMI	24,000,000	24,000,000	24,000,000	72,000,000
DFID	7,200,000			7,200,000
WHO + UNICEF	300,000	300,000	300,000	900,000
MACEPA	2,500,000			2,500,000
Private Sector	1,124,832	1,181,074	1,240,128	3,546,034
Total Funding Available	**63,124,832**	**53,981,074**	**54,540,128**	**171,646,034**
Zambia Malaria Funding Needed	95,377,364	103,107,665	160,521,267	359,006,296
Financial Gap	32,252,532	49,126,591	105,981,139	187,360,262

The total estimated funding for 2015 – 17 for malaria control activities is $359 million. If the Global Fund Concept Note is approved at the level requested, the total funding available will be approximately $368 million. Based upon the discussions so far, it is not expected that GRZ will receive the requested amount as there will have been requests for reductions to activities from the Global Fund. As a result, there will be a shortfall of funding during this period of time between the expected and actual amounts required for malaria control. This funding gap illustrates the need for a sustainability strategy by GRZ. By 2017, the difference between available and needed funding doubles despite the increase in the contribution by GRZ. This is due in part to the shift in the focus of funding by DFID and the uncertainty of funding from MACEPA. The costs in 2017 also increase significantly because of the need to replenish ITNs as a follow-up to the 2014 universal campaign, variable costs of IRS due to insecticide resistance, and expansion of ICCM to focus on high-burden areas. PMI may need to work with GRZ to convene partners to discuss the plan for targeted malaria prevention and control activities based on increasing costs and potentially decreasing financial support.

6.   PMI Goals, Targets and Indicators

The goal of PMI is to reduce malaria-associated mortality by 70% compared to pre-Initiative levels in the 15 original PMI countries. By the end of 2015, PMI will assist Zambia to achieve the following targets in populations at risk for malaria:

- >90% of households with a pregnant woman and/or children under five will own at least one ITN;
- 85% of children under five will have slept under an ITN the previous night;
- 85% of pregnant women will have slept under an ITN the previous night;
- 85% of houses in geographic areas targeted for IRS will have been sprayed;
- 85% of pregnant women and children under five will have slept under an ITN the previous night or in a house that has been sprayed with IRS in the last 6 months;
- 85% of women who have completed a pregnancy in the last two years will have received two or more doses of IPTp during that pregnancy; and
- 85% of government health facilities have ACTs available for treatment of uncomplicated malaria.

7.   Progress on Indicators to Date

At the national level, the MIS 2012 demonstrated a steady increase in intervention coverage and a continued reduction in the malaria parasite prevalence and severe anemia since 2006.

In 2012:
- Sixty-eight percent of households owned at least one ITN, compared to 64% in 2010 and 38% in 2006; 55% of households had at least one ITN per sleeping space, compared to 34% in 2010; and 73% of households were covered by at least one ITN or recent IRS, compared to 43% in 2006.
- Fifty-seven percent of children under age five years slept under an ITN the night before the survey (72% among households with at least one net), compared to 50% of these children in 2010 and 24% in 2006; and 58% of pregnant women reported sleeping under an ITN the previous night, compared to 46% in 2010 and 25% in 2006;
- Seventy-two percent of pregnant women reported taking two doses of IPTp during their last pregnancy, compared to 70% in 2010 and 59% in 2006;
- Eighty five percent of febrile children given an antimalarial drug received an ACT, compared to 76% in 2010 and 18% in 2006; and
- Fifteen percent of children ages 0–59 months had malaria parasitemia (microscopy), compared to 16% in 2010 and 22% in 2006

Table F: Indicator results of Malaria Indicator Surveys, 2006-2012				
Indicator	2006 MIS[1]	2008 MIS[2]	2010 MIS[3]	2012 MIS[4]
Percentage of households with at least one ITN	38	62	64	68
Percentage of households with at least one ITN per sleeping space	NA	33	34	55
Percentage of children under 5 years old who slept under an ITN the previous night	24	41	50	57
Percentage of pregnant women who slept under an ITN the previous night	25	43	46	58
Percentage of household members who slept under an ITN the previous night	19	34	42	49
Percentage of households covered by at least one ITN or recent IRS	43	68	73	73
Percentage of pregnant women who received two doses of intermittent preventive treatment during pregnancy	59	66	70	72
Percentage of febrile children under age five years with a reported finger stick for presumed diagnostic testing	NA	11	17	32
Among febrile children given antimalarial drug, the percentage that received ACT	18	30	76	85
Percentage of children ages 0–59 months with severe anemia (Hb<8 g/dl).	14	4	9	7
Percentage of children ages 0–59 months with malaria parasitemia (microscopy)	22	10	16	15

1. Zambia Ministry of Health, 2006. Zambia National Malaria Indicator Survey 2006. Lusaka, Zambia: Ministry of Health.
2. Zambia Ministry of Health, 2008. Zambia National Malaria Indicator Survey 2008. Lusaka, Zambia: Ministry of Health.
3. Zambia Ministry of Health, 2010. Zambia National Malaria Indicator Survey 2010. Lusaka, Zambia: Ministry of Health.
4. Zambia Ministry of Health, 2012. Zambia National Malaria Indicator Survey 2012. Lusaka, Zambia: Ministry of Health.

However, progress is not homogeneous throughout the country. Household ownership of at least one ITN ranges from 90% in Luapula Province to 52% in Western Province, and the percentage of households with at least one ITN per sleeping space varies from 83% in Luapula Province to 38% in Lusaka Province. Luapula's high ITN coverage likely contributed to a large drop in parasite prevalence. Lusaka parasite prevalence remains very low, and Copperbelt appears improved although HMIS data (malaria incidence rate of 402 per 1000 in 2013) is not consistent with a parasite prevalence of 4%. Four provinces had initial prevalence drops between 2006 and 2008 but have stagnated since (Southern, Central, Muchinga, and Northern). Eastern Province has the same parasitemia in 2012 as it did in 2006. Finally, two provinces (Western and North-Western) are headed backwards after initial success.

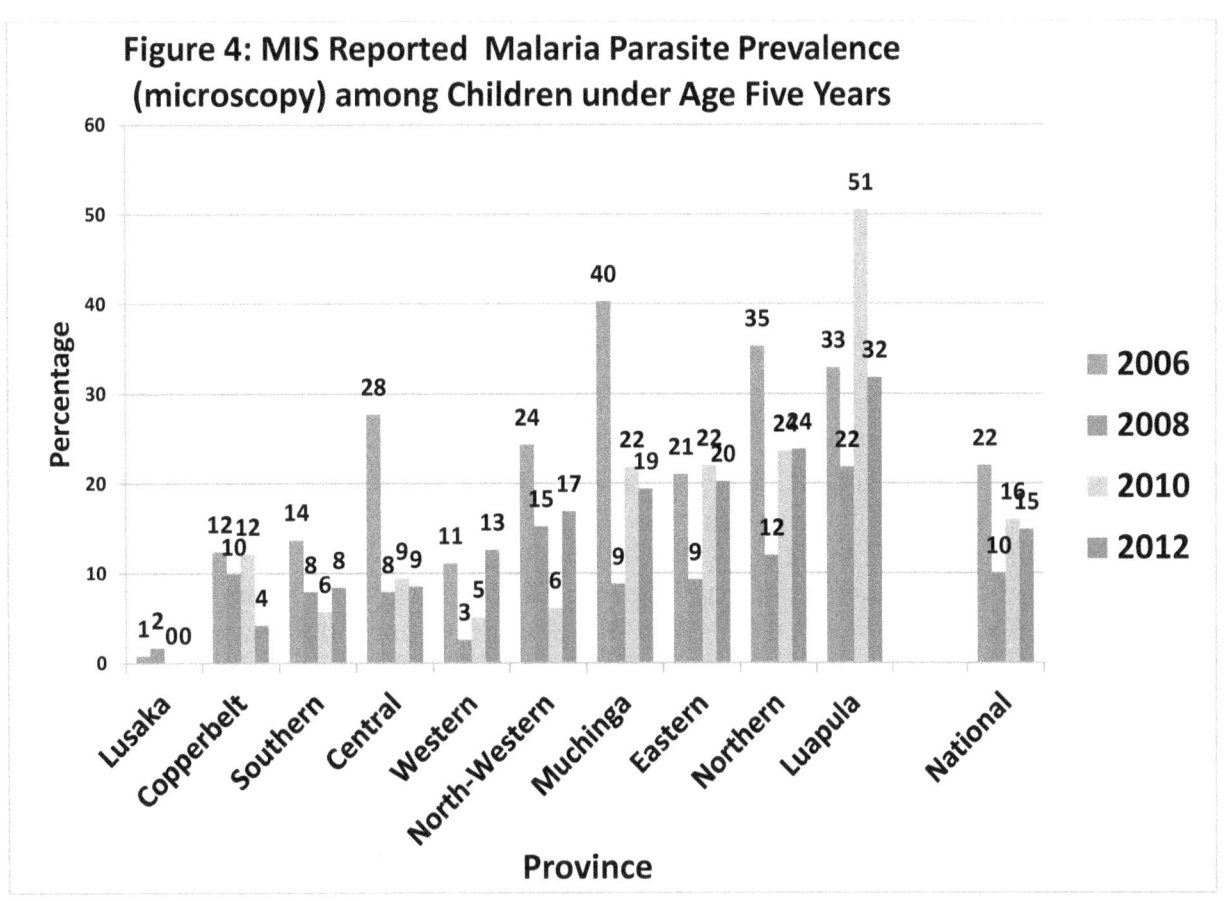

Figure 4: MIS Reported Malaria Parasite Prevalence (microscopy) among Children under Age Five Years

8. Other Relevant Evidence of Progress

The last nationwide health facility survey was in 2011. It provides insight into the preparedness of health facilities to deliver quality malaria services. The survey included 148 health facilities, of which 41 were hospitals, 38 were urban health centers, 39 were rural health centers and 30 were health posts. A total of 219 health workers were observed and 1,290 patients were assessed, of which 872 were suspected of having malaria. Key findings are:

- Testing for malaria was generally available; highest in hospitals (93%) and lowest in health posts (63%).
- The first-line drug also was available; most frequently in hospitals (95%) than in health posts (73%)
- Approximately one third of health workers had not received an in-service training in the last five years.
- Testing of suspected malaria reached 76% in children under five years of age.
- Seventy-three percent of "true positives" (after re-examination) received appropriate antimalarial treatment.

A program of enhanced surveillance and active community case detection and laboratory confirmation in Lusaka District has shown low levels of transmission. In 2011–2012, 395 index cases (17% of all cases of confirmed malaria) that had not traveled or had malaria in the month prior to testing were identified. A total of 5,795 persons associated with the index cases were tested in their homes or nearby homes. Only 91 (1.6%) of these neighborhood members were positive by RDT. The success of this program has been evident in the decision of the district health officials to take over funding in all 29 clinics in Lusaka District. This surveillance activity has also been implemented in selected clinics in seven other districts of Southern Province to help document elimination of malaria in five districts in Zambia by 2015.

9.   Challenges, Opportunities, and Threats

An important challenge for PMI continues to be the re-structuring of tasks traditionally carried out by the MOH to the MCDMCH at district level. During this MOP planning visit, PMI planned jointly with both the MOH and MCDMCH. During the last year, MCDMCH has recruited and filled a number of key positions at the central level. However, there are still a number of positions to be filled. In addition, the MCDMCH continues to work with MOH and other stakeholders to ensure that funds that were originally budgeted for the MOH are now being reflected in the MCDMCH budget. PMI's Resident Advisors (RAs) will follow the re-structuring process closely to ensure that there are no disruptions in PMI activities.

An important challenge for malaria control in Zambia, especially in an environment in which donor funds are stabilizing and even decreasing globally, is the heavy dependence on external funding. Capital and revolving costs have been mainly borne by donor partners since 2004. The MOH recognizes this dependence problem and has begun to increase its own funding for malaria control. The MOH procures all SP for IPTp and has included $27 million in its current budget (to be applied during 2014) to support several malaria activities. Additionally, in interviews with the MOP team, the Permanent of Secretary of Health reiterated that the $27 million will be a continuing contribution from the GRZ in the fight against malaria. DFID has been instrumental in working with the GRZ to increase governmental funding for malaria.

An additional challenge that continues to affects all interventions is the doubling of the official per diem rate. By some reports, depending on the type of health worker, the new per diem will be $100-$150 per day. The impact of this increase is being felt on activities funded under MOP 2013, as well as this MOP. The PMI in-country team and partners will be reviewing the effect this new directive will have on activities.

Zambia is moving into a new era of malaria control in which approaches and tools that have served well thus far to reach the current coverage levels will need to be revised to address the challenges of reaching the last mile. From dealing with late adopters of appropriate malaria behaviors to ensuring that commodities get to those hardest to reach, to developing monitoring and evaluation methods that provide accurate estimates in low prevalence settings, Zambia will need to maintain its gains while dealing with new scenarios to gain additional ground.

Intervention-specific challenges include the following:

ITNs

The intermittent nature of mass campaigns and the limited routine/continuous distribution channels has resulted in swings in coverage in Zambia. The household ownership of at least one ITN decreased in Western Province from 75% in 2010 to 52% in 2012. After the completion of the national mass LLIN campaign in 2014, it is critical that continuous/routine systems are in place and sufficient ITNs are procured to maintain high LLIN coverage. Full implementation of the additional channels will take time, thus another mass campaign is planned for 2017.

In 2012, Luapula Province had the highest ITN-to-sleeping-space ratio of at least one-to-one at 83%, under-five use of 78%, and pregnant women use of 82%. Yet, Luapula Province had the highest percentage of parasitemia (32%) and severe anemia (12%). One factor likely contributing to this persistent high malaria burden is documented *Anopheles* resistance to pyrethroid insecticides. In response and with the support of DFID funding, focal IRS will be conducted in Luapula using organophosphates during 2014 and 2015 spray seasons. Another factor could be inconsistent net utilization.

IRS

Continued IRS challenges include reduced donor and partner support to IRS. With the ending of World Bank IRS support in 2012, PMI is the only donor supporting IRS in the country. Mining companies, mainly in the Copperbelt Province, continue to support IRS albeit on a limited scale and confined to the areas in which they operate. Other challenges include inadequate supervision at the district level, inadequate storage facilities, and poor store room stock-keeping practices. PMI continues to focus on the 20 old boundary districts and covers all IRS associated costs. Non-PMI-supported IRS did not take place last year due to a lack of insecticide. The MOH committed significant funding to IRS in 2014 and appeared to be moving forward with the procurement of US$10M of Actellic CS for the 2014 spray season. However, the process was delayed leading to concerns being raised about whether the insecticide would be delivered on time. Furthermore, it is unknown if funding for IRS implementation will be available.

Currently, government funding to the districts is inadequate to enable them to implement recommendations made during environmental inspections; storage facilities have limited space for keeping of all IRS commodities; and soak pits are not fully secured at some locations. A unique opportunity exists for assessing the impact of targeted IRS through a controlled trial. A study has been proposed to investigate variation in parasite prevalence in LLIN-protected populations using different IRS coverage strategies.

Focal IRS will be conducted in Luapula Province with DFID funding using organophosphates during 2014 and 2015 spray seasons. However, there isn't any commitment from DFID to continue supporting IRS beyond the 2015 spray season.

Insecticide resistance is a major threat to the effectiveness of the IRS program in Zambia, as resistance to DDT, pyrethroids, and carbamates has been detected in several parts of Zambia.

Changing to alternative insecticides such as long-acting organophosphates increases program costs substantially. Resistance to pyrethroids also raises concern about ITN effectiveness, given that pyrethroids are the only insecticide currently available for use in ITNs.

MIP

Sulfadoxine-pyrimethamine (SP) resistance continues to be a threat for IPTp, and a review of the current evidence on SP IPTp efficacy resulted in an updated WHO policy in 2012. The NMCP has updated their policy to align with the WHO policy. Updating of the IPTp policy has necessitated retraining of healthcare workers and updating BCC materials.

A PMI-funded study of SP IPTp efficacy in Mansa, Zambia was completed in 2013. This study found a 26% parasitological failure rate for IPTp-SP relative to the moderate 61% prevalence of the quintuple mutant among pregnant women with asymptomatic malaria parasitemia. The threat of SP resistance looms, and continuous resistance monitoring is needed especially in light of the emergence of the sextuple mutation, but IPTp-SP seems to retain some degree of efficacy in Mansa. Although the study cannot be generalized for Zambian women nation-wide, this provides evidence that IPTp is still effective in the study population of Zambian women.

A challenge in SP IPTp uptake is the cultural practice of not revealing a pregnancy until a woman shows obvious physical signs of being pregnant or late in the second trimester. This results in late presentation to ANC clinic and missed opportunities to provide IPTp. In addition, cultural and knowledge barriers resulting in decreased uptake of IPTp will require continued BCC regarding IPTp. Also, as found in a qualitative evaluation of barriers to receiving SP for IPTp, performed at the end of 2011 in two rural districts within each of three provinces with high malaria prevalence, many women believe only one ANC visit is needed, thus impacting the number of IPTp doses received.

Another challenge for reducing MIP is the use of high-dose folic acid in FANC in Zambia as it reduces the efficacy of SP for IPTp. Pregnant women are routinely given 5 mg folate tablets as a part of FANC. Because the tablets are cheaper if bought in bulk, 5mg tablets are the only strength of folate purchased and these tablets are the standard folate tablets given to all women at ANC whether for prenatal supplementation or for folate deficiency. The WHO recommends 0.4 mcg as the prenatal supplemental dose. This low dose contrasts with the 5mg dose given to pregnant women in Zambia.

Case Management – Diagnostics

Without a national malaria diagnostics QA/QC framework, there continues to be confusion over roles and responsibilities at the various levels on the health system. This has been exacerbated further by the re-structuring and devolution of tasks traditionally carried out by the MOH/NMCC to the MCDMCH at district level.

The doubling of the daily subsistence allowance for staff as required by the MOH has slowed implementation of training and supervision activities, decreasing the number of health facilities that can be reached annually. QA for RDTs is especially needed as field visits have uncovered inappropriate retesting within two weeks with RDTs after positive results.

Case Management – Treatment

During the 2014 malaria commodities quantification exercise, it was noted that there were significant discrepancies between the number of malaria cases reported by districts through the HMIS, and the ACT consumption reported by Essential Medicines Malaria Logistics improvement Program (EMLIP) districts. For example, Kaloma District in Southern Province reported 5,901 malaria cases through the HMIS between October , 2012 and September 30, 2013, but the number of ACT treatments reported consumed through EMLIP was 62,581. The reason for this discrepancy is under investigation. Possible reasons include under-reporting of cases through the HMIS, not reporting cases treated by CHWs, buildup of ACT stocks at health facility level, and pilfering of ACTs. In February 2014 the Drug Enforcement Commission did recover a large suitcase filled with commodities including ACTs from a public bus.

Although iCCM has the potential to expand access to malaria case management, the trainings have often outpaced the needed logistical support. Many trained CHWs are not fully functional due to the lack of malaria commodities. Malaria commodities must flow through heath facilities to CHWs. If the facilities are in short supply, providers are less likely to release malaria commodities to CHWs.

Case Management – Pharmaceutical Management

With growth in HIV, TB, Malaria and other programs over past years, storage space at Medical Stores Limited (MSL) has become one of the major constraints in achieving health outcomes. Most health facilities cannot guarantee safe storage of health commodities due to inadequate storage space. To address these challenges, USAID is currently supporting outsourcing of extra storage space at the central level. Over the past years, the USAID has procured prefabricated storage units using PEPFAR funds which have been installed at six different sites. This has helped to mitigate storage space issues at health facilities. Furthermore, following the policy directive by the MOH to ensure last mile distribution, the USAID is supporting the GRZ with construction of two regional warehouses (Hubs) in Mansa and Luanshya districts.

Delayed disbursement of government funding for procurement of health commodities in general and malarial commodities in particular is a recurrent problem in Zambia. This has resulted in delayed procurements leading to stockouts. In 2013, the GRZ allocated $24 million for procurement of malaria commodities but only $15 million was spent. However, malaria commodities continues to receive donor support and this has helped to mitigate stockouts and improve stock availability at both central and service delivery point (SDP) level. The GRZ has increased budgetary allocation for procurement of malaria commodities from $24 million in 2013 to $27 million in 2014 and they hope to increase it further to $30 million in 2015.

BCC

Zambia faces a dichotomy of advanced malaria control in the Southern Province, while dealing with upticks in malaria cases in the Copperbelt, North-Western, and Luapula Provinces. The approach to BCC activities must also be tailored to address this. As Zambia advances in its control of malaria in the South the behavioral issues it will encounter will be more and more complex and likely demand further investment to resolve them; while on the other hand, scaling up in areas of increasing incidence requires a different approach. For example, the recent undertaking of universal LLIN coverage campaigns throughout the country raises challenges to ensure that increased coverage and access results in increased use by focusing BCC activities for continued use in some populations, newly-adopted use in other populations, while combating complacency of use yet in others.

Monitoring and Evaluation

Areas in Zambia where malaria is declining pose an important challenge to M&E activities. As malaria prevalence declines, standard household surveys will become less and less useful to detect, with appropriate accuracy, changes in malaria population-based indicators. Other methods for monitoring trends and impact will need to be devised and implemented. More attention and resources will need to be paid to HMIS as it will become the backbone information source as prevalence declines.

The HMIS has been migrated to District Health Information System (DHIS2) software. This allows for internet access to malaria data.
Although improving, problems with timeliness and completeness of HMIS data remain. Most health facilities still use paper forms to record and forwarded to the districts. Switching to rapid reporting with phones could be a way to improve timeliness and accuracy.

The utilization of data for decision making remains sub-optimal and feedback to end users is still a problem. MCDMCH has hired an epidemiologist on the malaria team which provides an opportunity to expand data analysis and use. The addition of FETP residents will also provide support.

Health Systems Strengthening and Capacity Building

Significant progress has been made regarding the reorganization of the public health sector. However, challenges still remain with regard to division of malaria-related activities between the two ministries. The staff from the malaria unit at the MCDMCH are not currently co-located with the MOH staff, making co-ordination between the two ministries challenging. The MOH/NMCC will need to coordinate with the MCDMCH on malaria service delivery from the district level down. Most of the GRZ funding for malaria, including funding for implementation at district level, is channeled through the MOH, making planning for implementation activities such as IRS through the MCDMCH challenging.

Recently unstaffed positions at the MOH/NMCC include the Case Management Officer and the Chief Entomologist. The MOH has stated that filling these positions are a priority.

10.   PMI Support Strategy

PMI's support strategy in Zambia is to complement funding from other donors and focus on NMCP priorities that are not addressed by other funding sources. PMI also provides targeted technical assistance. In the recent past, PMI has supported IRS, ITN distribution through ANC and EPI clinics, and procurement and distribution of antimalarials and RDTs. In all instances, PMI is not the sole donor but works with partners to ensure that all necessary resources are available for the country's needs. This strategy has meant PMI is involved, to some degree, in almost all aspects of the malaria program and is often a key player in resolving unexpected problems because of the flexibility of PMI resources.

PMI will continue to provide technical assistance to NMCP at the national and sub-national levels through USAID, CDC, and partners to meet the goals of the National Malaria Strategic Plan (NMSP). This support is evident in activities such as:
- updating the Malaria Case Management policy in Zambia;
- contributions to the Global Fund Concept Note;
- recommendations for targeting IRS based upon universal coverage of ITNs; and
- routine data analysis of HMIS data for malaria to identify trends and areas that require investigation to determine reasons for changes in malaria patterns.

PMI plans to continue assistance to the MOH/NMCC and will also focus on building the capacity of MCDMCH as they expand their activities and responsibilities within the NMCP.

OPERATIONAL PLAN

1.   Insecticide-Treated Nets

NMCP/PMI Objectives

Zambia's Strategic Plan calls for universal net coverage, which is defined as "ensuring all sleeping spaces in targeted households are covered by an ITN." The revised NMSP (2011–2016) makes universal ITN coverage the main strategy for achieving sustained vector control for all people at risk of malaria infection in the country. IRS will be added to ITNs in densely populated areas with insecticide resistance and high malaria burden.

In order to achieve universal coverage, a number of delivery methods have been adopted. These include free mass distribution of ITNs and routine distribution to pregnant women and children under-five years of age through ANC and EPI clinics. As a result of these efforts, the percentage of homes with at least one ITN increased from 38% in 2006 to 68% in 2012. In addition, the number of households with an ITN-to-sleeping space ratio of one-to-one increased from 32% in 2008 to 55% in 2012. Despite the progress, ITN coverage remains below the country's universal coverage target. In addition, the MIS 2012 showed that ITN coverage also varies across provinces, ranging from 52% in Western, to 90% in Luapula.

To address falling coverage levels in some provinces, the NMCP planned a national mass ITN campaign for 2013/2014. The initial estimated ITN need was 8,998,200, based on a population of 14,762,300 in 2014, one ITN per 1.8 population, and an additional 10% buffer. This total was decreased by about 600,000 ITNs when a consensus was reached not to target the Lusaka urban population, where the malaria risk is very low. The GRZ has received financial and technical support for the mass campaign from a number of stakeholders, including the Global Fund, PMI, DFID, UNICEF, WHO, MACEPA, and others.

The NMCP has a target of 80% use of ITNs by children under five years and pregnant women by 2016. ITN use in children under five increased from 24% in 2006 to 57% in 2012. Eastern Province reported the highest under-five use at 80% and Lusaka had the lowest at 40%. The under-five utilization was 68% nationally in households with at least one ITN. Fifty-eight percent of pregnant women reported sleeping under an ITN in 2012, ranging from 39% in Copperbelt to 89% in Eastern.

Progress during the last year

The mass campaign started in Western Province in 2013 with support from DFID. World Vision conducted a door-to-door campaign distributing 770,000 ITNs to cover every sleeping space. The LLIN need, based on official population figures, was underestimated at 591,000 nets. Copperbelt Province also conducted a mass campaign in 2013 with support from World Bank, PMI, and World Vision. PMI contributed 652,100 ITNs to the campaign in Copperbelt. Mass campaigns also occurred in rural districts of Lusaka Province during 2013.

The remaining seven provinces will conduct mass ITN campaigns beginning in June 2014. PMI is supporting Luapula Province and Global Fund/UNDP is funding the other six provinces. PMI has partnered with World Vision in Luapula Province. PMI will supply sufficient ITNs to assure universal coverage and World Vision will fund the distribution costs with private donor funding. The ITN need for Luapula based on the national census is 669,900. However, the final number will be based on the household census of sleeping spaces.

PMI also supports routine ITN distribution systems in Zambia. Every district received ITNs for ANC distribution totaling 446,700 nets. In addition, 100,200 ITNs were distributed through PEPFAR programming, and another 61,200 through the Anglican Church via community based distribution in Western Province, as part of the Zambia –Angola cross border initiative.

The PMI supported a situational analysis and stakeholders NetCalc workshop in Zambia in January 2014. The analysis concluded that ANC/EPI channels were not sufficient to replace worn out nets over time, and additional channels were required. After reviewing different scenarios, a consensus was reached on adding primary schools and community-based distributions to the existing ANC/EPI channels. NetCalc shows that these four channels can maintain LLIN ownership levels at 90%. PMI supported the development of a draft Zambia Continuous/Routine Distribution Guideline and will begin to pilot the expanded channels in Luapula in 2015.

PMI supported operational research to examine the durability of ITNs to guide decisions about net replacement. ITNs distributed in 2011 in Northern and Luapula Provinces are being tracked and examined for structural integrity and insecticide content through December 2013. Data was collected by Peace Corps Volunteers at the provincial and local levels. The data is being analyzed and final results are expected in late 2014.

Commodity gap analysis

The ITN population-based gap analysis (Table G) is based on the official population figures for Zambia, minus the estimated Lusaka urban population. The calculation is based on an estimate of one ITN per 1.8 persons, plus 10% to account for inaccuracies in population projections. As noted previously, the population numbers underestimate the population by as much as 30% when a household census is carried out to determine sleeping spaces. Thus the "surpluses" in 2014 and 2015 are not likely to be real.

Table G: Gap Analysis for ITNs 2014-2016			
Calendar Year	2014	2015	2016
Total Population	14,621,790	15,031,200	15,452,074
Total Targeted Population Mass Campaign*	13,623,210	13,998,669	14,384,436
LLIN Need	8,325,295	8,554,742	8,790,489
Viable LLINs**			
2013	2,690,068	1,681,293	
2014		5,656,240	3,535,150
2015			1,200,000
Partner Commitments			
Routine			
MOH		200,000	300,000
PMI	388,055	800,000	400,000
DFID	200,000	360,000	0
Global Fund		0	857,436
Campaign			
MOH	200,000		
PMI	1,200,000		400,000***
DFID	271,945		
Global Fund	4,810,300		
Total Funded	7,070,300	1,360,000	1,957,436
Total LLINs Available	9,760,368	8,697,533	6,292,586
Annual LLIN Surplus/Gap	**1,435,073**	**142,791**	**-2,497,903**
*Does not include Lusaka Urban			
**Decay rates = 8% 1st year 20% 2nd year, and 50% 3rd year			
***400,000 LLINs will be procured in 2016 for 2017 mass campaign and are not available in 2016			

Plans and justification

With FY 2015 funding, PMI will focus on the procurement and distribution of ITNs to maintain a supply of nets for continuous/routine distribution through ANC/EPI, primary school, and community channels. PMI will provide technical assistance for the roll out of primary school and community distribution, as well as strategies for care and maintenance of nets. In addition, PMI will continue to monitor the durability of ITNs distributed during the mass campaign. In order to maximize ITN usage, PMI will continue to support BCC activities, prioritizing local over national activities.

Proposed activities with FY 2015 funding ($3,700,000)

- Procurement and distribution of approximately 800,000 ITNs for free continuous/routine distribution and 2017 mass campaign, ($3,400,000);

- Support the roll out of additional continuous/routine distribution channels for sustaining high ITN coverage, as well as strategies for care and repair of nets, in four high burden provinces. ($300,000).

- Monitor attrition/survivorship and physical integrity of ITNs following mass campaign. (see M&E section)

- CDC technical assistance for routine monitoring of net durability (see M&E section)

- Support BCC activities to increase consistent utilization of ITNs. (see BCC section)

2.   Indoor Residual Spraying

NMCP/PMI Objectives

The Zambian NMCP aims to provide access to evidence-based vector control to 100% of households and persons at risk in targeted areas by 2016. The NMCP's goal is to achieve and sustain universal ITN coverage in conjunction with a focal, data-driven approach to prioritize IRS. The NMCP views IRS as an important additional vector control method for reducing transmission and managing resistance in areas with documented resistance to pyrethroids and high malaria incidence. IRS is recognized as the only intervention available to manage insecticide resistance through rotation among different classes of WHOPES-approved insecticides, making entomological monitoring an indispensable component of an evidence-based resistance management program.

Progress during the last year

PMI supported the NMCP IRS operations in 20 PMI focus districts (seven in Eastern Province; five in Muchinga Province; eight in Northern Province). Approximately   structures were sprayed, out of the targeted 529,564 (81.7% coverage) protecting 1,842,821 people (approximately 10% of the Zambian population). PMI support to NMCP IRS programs included training, geocoding, and procurement of insecticides and personal protection equipment. Equipment procured included: 218 spray pumps, 64 repair kits with 675 #8002 nozzles, and personal protective equipment (671 hard hats; 1,471 overalls; 865 gum boots, 1,811 pairs of gloves, 37,600 respirator masks). The payment system for spray operators in 15 districts was improved through mobile payment and off-the-counter bank payment. In January 2014 PMI expanded its support to an additional nine districts in two provinces with DFID funding, bringing the total to 29 districts (total of 40 districts following the Government of Zambia's recent district re-demarcation exercise).

The IRS program was conducted in compliance with United States Government's USAID Regulation 216, Zambia Environmental Management Act cap 204, No 12 of 2011, and USAID Initial and Supplemental Environmental Assessments and Pesticide Evaluation Report and Safer Use Action Plan and its amendments. During October–December 2013, pre- and mid-spray environmental compliance inspections were conducted in the 20 old boundary districts, as was random inspection of houses sprayed to check for quality of messages to homeowners after the spray. End-of-day clean-ups and triple rinsing practice to check for liquid waste management checks were also carried out. Post-spray inventories in all 20 old boundary districts were conducted during February–March 2014; 17 districts carried out clean-ups at time of inspection; 3 districts (Mbala, Chilubi & Chama) finished later. An insecticide inventory verified good stock control in all sites. Micro-planning meetings were conducted in all the 20 old boundary districts in May 2014.

During the 2013 spray season, organophosphates were used across the whole country. Residual efficacy testing was conducted in three sentinel sites (Katete, Kasama, Isoka) in the three PMI-supported provinces. Tests in Katete recorded 100% mortality after 24 hours exposure of the vectors to insecticide. However, the mud surface tested in Isoka and Kasama yielded 78% and 63% mortality respectively after 24 hours of exposure. One house out the two houses with mud surface in Isoka recorded mortality less than 100%, however, in Kasama, both mud houses recorded mortality less than 100%.

Insecticide resistance to available IRS chemicals continued to pose a threat to the IRS program. With PMI assistance, the MOH/NMCC developed a more complete map of insecticide resistance in the country. Previous insecticide resistance surveys have reported resistance in the two major malaria vector species; *An. gambiae* and *An. funestus*. A recent survey conducted in 2013-2014 reported *An. gambiae* resistance to pyrethroids throughout Zambia. Resistance to bendiocarb (a carbamate) was found, particularly in areas of Luapula and Northern provinces. DDT resistance was also widespread. *An. funestus* was reported to be largely susceptible to DDT but resistant to pyrethroids throughout the country. *An. funestus* populations in the Eastern province were shown to be resistant to bendiocarb. However, all vector species were found to be susceptible to organophosphates. The NMCP, with support from PMI, drafted an Insecticide Resistance Management Plan that calls for periodic scheduled rotation of insecticides used in the IRS program, including DDT. The NMCP plans to use DDT in some areas of the country in the 2015 or 2016 IRS spray season.

The MOH committed significant funding to IRS in 2014. With funding from the Zambian government, the NMCP initiated the procurement of $10 million worth of organophosphates for use in the 2014 spray season in non-PMI supported areas.

Procurement of a pre-fabricated insectary to be stationed at the NMCP was initiated with an expected delivery of 90 days (September, 2014). Three additional sentinel sites for routine entomological monitoring were established in the DFID funded areas, bringing the total number of PMI supported sentinel sites to six. Baseline entomological data was collected in DFID-supported districts from February–March, 2014. In addition, biochemical assays were conducted on vector mosquitoes to determine metabolic mechanisms of resistance in May 2014.

The IRS TWG proposed changes in IRS procedures for planning and monitoring in order to effectively target areas to be sprayed, with recommendations to define target areas based on insecticide resistance, high incidence rate, high population/high structure density, and accessibility. These changes are planned to be implemented in PMI supported areas in the 2014 spray season (September 2014–December 2014). In addition, satellite-based enumeration was implemented in Luapula and Central provinces.

Previous efforts to identify a local recycling company that could recycle empty Actellic bottles into appropriate products were unsuccessful. In 2014, a decision was made to have the Actellic bottles recycled in South Africa, and a local company in Lusaka was identified to coordinate recycling. Approximately 78,000 plastic bottles collected from the 2012/13 spray season were baled at the company in Lusaka in readiness for transportation to South Africa for recycling. The recycled plastic will be used to make products such as chairs and dust bins.

Table H : IRS Coverage and Insecticide Use 2011-2015					
Calendar Year	Number of Districts Sprayed	Insecticide Used	Number of Structures Sprayed	Coverage Rate	Population Protected
2011	35	Carbamate, Organophospahte,Pyrethroid	1,200,000	83%	6,200,000
2012	20	Carbamates (FICAM®), Organophosphate (Actellic ®)	460,303	86%	1,710,833
2013	20	Organophosphate (Actellic ®)	432,398	81%	1,842,821
2014*	40	Organophosphate (Actellic ®)	472,000	-	-
2015**	40	Organophosphate (Actellic ®)	450,000	-	-

2014 and 2015 targets include DFID funded Districts
*Represents targets based on the revised 2014 IRS work plan
**Represents revised projected targets

Figure 5. Insecticide resistance status

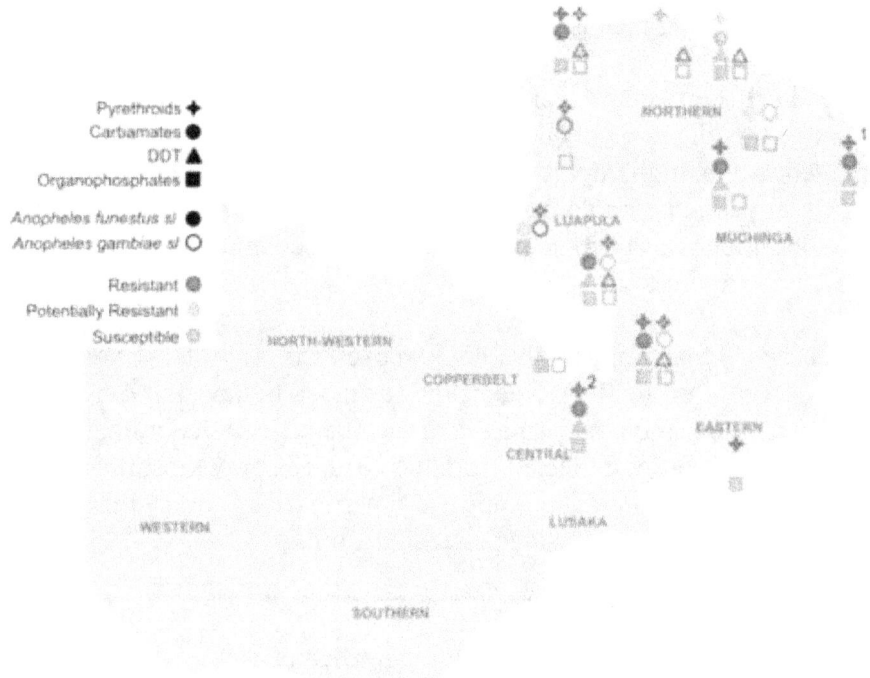

Figure 6: PMI and DFID Supported Districts - Old boundary districts

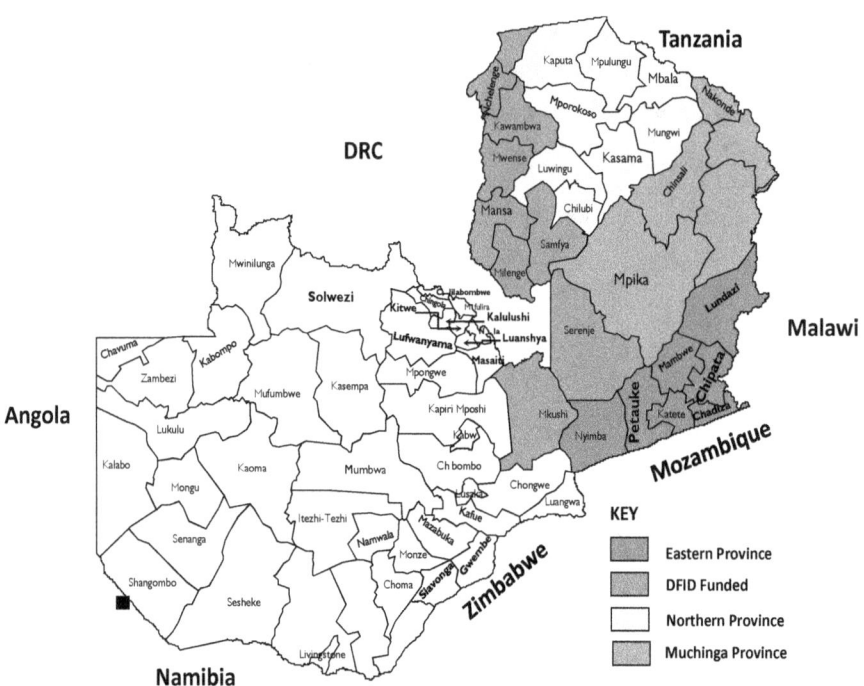

Plans and justification

PMI will cover the cost of IRS in the 20 old boundary districts in five provinces: Central (2 districts), Eastern, Luapula, Muchinga, and Northern. Approximately 450,000 structures will be targeted protecting, more than two million people. The actual number of household/structures sprayed will depend on the cost of insecticides selected, the cost of implementation and the incidence of the disease in the district.

Planned activities also include expanded insecticide resistance monitoring and management, entomological monitoring, and support of environmental assessments. Specific activities include: pre-season environmental compliance inspection; collection of empty plastics bottles generated from the previous spray campaign; support to rehabilitation of IRS facilities such as soak pits, shower rooms & change rooms; support for MOH/NMCC and MCDMCH to conduct training of trainers for spray operators; preparing a "Letter Report" for environmental compliance; launching spray operations in all the 40 districts; carrying out periodic testing of vector population for phenotypic resistance; carrying out pre-spray vector population density determination in PMI supported sentinel sites; supporting NMCP teams to carry out monitoring and supervision during IRS implementation; procurement of organophosphate insecticide, spray pumps, PPE, and other IRS commodities.

PMI supports the MOH policy to rotate the insecticide used for IRS, based on evidence of vector resistance to insecticides. The recommendation from the Insecticide Resistance Management Technical Advisory Committee is to rotate to DDT in 2015 or 2016 in selected districts. PMI will explore the feasibility of using DDT in the Eastern province.

The NMCP is using other partners for small-scale larviciding projects in Lusaka and has not asked PMI for support.

Proposed activities with FY 2015 funding ($8,168,700)

- Procure insecticides and other IRS supplies/equipment for spraying up to 450,000 structures in 40 districts, inclusive of districts previously supported by DFID, pending the insecticides selected and associated costs. Support environmental monitoring and environmental assessment, to include use of DDT, organophosphates, or carbamates. ($6,170,500);

- Train spray operators, supervisors, and store keepers; monitoring and evaluation; BCC for IRS; pesticide storage; waste disposal; and pay for spray operations in 40 PMI-funded districts; ($1,674,000);

- Support entomological monitoring in at least 40 PMI supported districts, assisting with operations of the new insectary; work with NMCP to coordinate and facilitate the collection of entomological information, its analysis and interpretation to inform decision making in targeting vector control and pesticide selection for IRS; and continue insecticide resistance management ($300,000); and

- CDC technical assistance for entomological monitoring and insecticide resistance ($24,200).

3.   Malaria in Pregnancy

NMCP/PMI Objectives

The NMCP has set a goal that all pregnant women attending ANC clinics receive at least two doses of SP for IPTp by 2016. In 2013, an initial attempt was made to align the national policy on IPTp with the recently updated WHO policy on IPTp. The national policy is now for pregnant women to receive SP IPTp at every monthly opportunity. IPTp is given at least one month apart up to the time of delivery with the first dose starting after 16 weeks of gestation. Technical working groups meet regularly to move the Malaria in Pregnancy agenda forward in Zambia. These groups include representatives from the MOH, MCDMCH, and various malaria and reproductive health partners including PMI.

PMI has supported three main strategies to address malaria in pregnancy: IPTp, ITNs, and case management. IPTp is discussed in detail below. ITNs were procured and distributed to pregnant women through ANCs and universal coverage campaigns (see ITN section for details). PMI also supported appropriate case management of malaria in pregnancy through trainings of healthcare workers on malaria diagnosis and treatment guidelines (see Case Management section for details).

Progress during the last year

Focused antenatal care (FANC) is a comprehensive prenatal care package provided to pregnant women at ANC clinics that includes care related to malaria such as providing SP for IPTp, providing an ITN at the first ANC visit, and educating pregnant women on the importance of seeking care immediately for fever.

A FANC rapid assessment, conducted in two districts per province in 2011, reported barriers to IPTp coverage being primarily lack of training in FANC in the last two years (66%), stock outs of SP (64% of facilities surveyed had SP stock outs in the last quarter), and late first-time attendance to ANC clinic (60%). Furthermore, the MIS 2012 found that women in rural areas had lower coverage of at least two doses of IPTp than women in urban areas (78% v 69%). FY 2014 activities focused on addressing these issues.

FANC training and supervision is provided to healthcare workers via clinical care teams (CCTs) present in all districts and provinces nationwide. These teams consist of staff that are already part of the health system, namely a clinical care supervisor and a CHW coordinator. Provincial-level CCTs supervise and train district-level CCTs and health workers at district-level facilities. District-level CCTs train and supervise health workers at the local facility level. PMI has supported the malaria in pregnancy component of training for the CCTs. As of the end of the second quarter of FY 2014, 324 health workers targeted in 27 districts across all provinces have received training in FANC.

Because the availability of SP is critical for IPTp, PMI has continued to invest in EMLIP to improve distribution of malaria commodities (see Treatment and Pharmaceutical Management section) and to prevent stockouts of malaria commodities like SP in ANCs. Availability of SP has since improved due to these investments.

SP resistance continues to be monitored as a threat to the efficacy IPTp. A PMI-funded study by Tan et al.[1] of the efficacy of SP for IPTp in Mansa, Zambia was completed in 2013. This study found a 26% parasitological failure rate for IPTp-SP relative to the moderate 61% prevalence of the quintuple mutant among pregnant women with asymptomatic malaria parasitemia. The threat of SP resistance looms, and continuous resistance monitoring is needed especially in light of the emergence of the sextuple mutation, but IPTp-SP seems to retain some degree of efficacy in Mansa. Although the study cannot be generalized for Zambian women nation-wide, this provides evidence that IPTp is still effective in the study population of Zambian women.

National BCC efforts for MIP are now part of a larger integrated campaign on maternal health and nutrition that disseminates messages through national radio and television spots encouraging early prenatal care, use of nets during pregnancy, and the importance of IPTp.

Community BCC efforts focus around educating and training Safe Motherhood Action Groups (SMAGs), where they are present, on MIP and other aspects of ANC. Other community BCC activities related to MIP were also supported by PMI in FY 2014 (see BCC section). A PMI partner has been implementing an integrated community-based communications initiative called "Champion Communities" focusing on promotion of malaria prevention, diagnosis, appropriate treatment, since 2011. The objectives of the initiative include having all pregnant women in the community attend ANC early and receive the recommended doses of IPTp. The initiative is being implemented in 8 districts and 131 communities across four higher malaria burden provinces.

The initiative has recorded impressive results, with the proportion of pregnant women who attended ANC increasing from 60% to 93% and the proportion of eligible pregnant women who received IPTp increasing from 57% to 95% in the targeted communities.

---

[1] Tan et al. *Malaria Journal* 2014, 13:227
http://www.malariajournal.com/content/13/1/227

Table I: Programmatic-based Gap Analysis for SP 2014-2016			
SP Needs and Contributions	**2014**	**2015**	**2016**
Estimated population	14,621,790	15,031,200	15,452,074
Expected pregnancies	760,334	781,622	803,508
Number of pregnant women attending ANC (97%)	737,524	758,174	779,403
Total SP needs (Tablets)	5,752,146	5,913,759	6,079,344
Commitments			
SP from MOH (Tablets)	6,300,000	0	0
SP from PMI (Tablets)	0	0	0
SP from Global Fund	0	0	0
SP from other sources	0	0	0
Total Funded	6,300,000	0	0
Previous year surplus	14,000,000	14,547,854	8,634,095
Annual SP Surplus/Gap	14,547,854	8,634,095	2,554,751

Assumptions: Population growth is estimated at 2.8% and based on 2010 population census data. Approximately 5.2% of national population is pregnant mothers. Total antenatal attendance estimated at 97% in 2014. 95.0% of pregnant mothers attending antenatal clinics will receive 1st IPTp dose, 80% will receive 2nd IPTp dose and 65% will receive the 3rd IPTp dose. 20% of the total antenatal attendances visit the health facilities at the right time (4th month of pregnancy) and are likely to receive the 4th IPTp dose in 2014. This assumption was applied for 2014 to 2016.

Plans and justification

The NMCP goal of 100% coverage with at least two doses of SP for IPTp was set based on the high average baseline coverage of 70% found in the MIS 2010. In spite of high coverage, there is a disparity of coverage between urban and rural women. The strategy to increase IPTp coverage includes targeting rural areas.

To strengthen delivery of care related to prevention and treatment of MIP, and in light of the updated NMCP IPTp policy, PMI will continue to support supervision and training of health center clinical staff in FANC in the updated policies through CCTs. The newly-trained district-level CCTs will focus their initial training and supervisory visits on rural facilities.

Because cultural and knowledge barriers resulting in decreased uptake of IPTp will require continued BCC regarding IPTp, PMI has and will continue to make investments in BCC to prevent MIP (see BCC section). A knowledge, attitudes, and practices survey planned for 2015 should give insight on the impact of our investments in BCC to prevent MIP.

To improve patient knowledge and demand for prevention and treatment of malaria in pregnancy, PMI will continue to support national- and community-level BCC activities, with an emphasis on local BCC activities such as SMAGs in rural areas.

Proposed activities with FY 2014 funding ($450,000)

- Train provincial-level, and district-level CCTs in four high-malaria-burden provinces on the updated NMCP IPTp guidelines, ($450,000);

- National and community BCC efforts for MIP will include messages through national and local radio, national television spots, and SMAGs encouraging timely ANC attendance, encouraging ANC visits during pregnancy, use of nets during pregnancy, and updated IPTp recommendations (see BCC section).

4.   Case Management

Diagnostics

NMCP/PMI Objectives

The Guidelines for the Diagnosis and Treatment of Malaria in Zambia (Fourth Edition 2014) are aligned with the revised 2010 WHO recommendations on universal diagnostic testing for malaria. The NMSP Strategic Plan 2011-2016 diagnostic objective is to ensure all suspected malaria cases receive parasitological confirmation by 2016. Parasitological confirmation is done by examining either a blood smear/slide by microscopy or malaria RDT. Antimalarial treatment based on a clinical diagnosis should only be considered when a parasitological diagnosis is not immediately available.

Microscopy should be used where there is a well-functioning laboratory with staff well-trained in malaria diagnostics. RDTs are to be used in health facilities where there is no microscopy or no well-trained laboratory staff, when a laboratory is closed or too busy to handle the work load and at the community level by CHWs trained in iCCM.

Progress during the last year

The NMCP, PMI, and partners have invested in three key areas related to malaria diagnostics: 1) procurement and distribution of diagnostic commodities; 2) training of clinical and laboratory personnel in the use of these diagnostic tools; and 3) training of national, provincial, and district level staff in providing outreach training and supportive supervision (OTSS) for quality assurance of malaria diagnostics.

This investment is having an impact. The percentage of children with fever that reported having a heel or finger stick increased from 17% (MIS 2010) to 32% (MIS 2012). The HMIS confirms progress in diagnostics. Fifty-two percent of reported malaria cases were confirmed in 2013, compared with 31% in 2010, and 69% were confirmed nationally in the first quarter of 2014

(HMIS). In 2013, the percent confirmed ranged from 33% in Western Province to 78% in Southern.

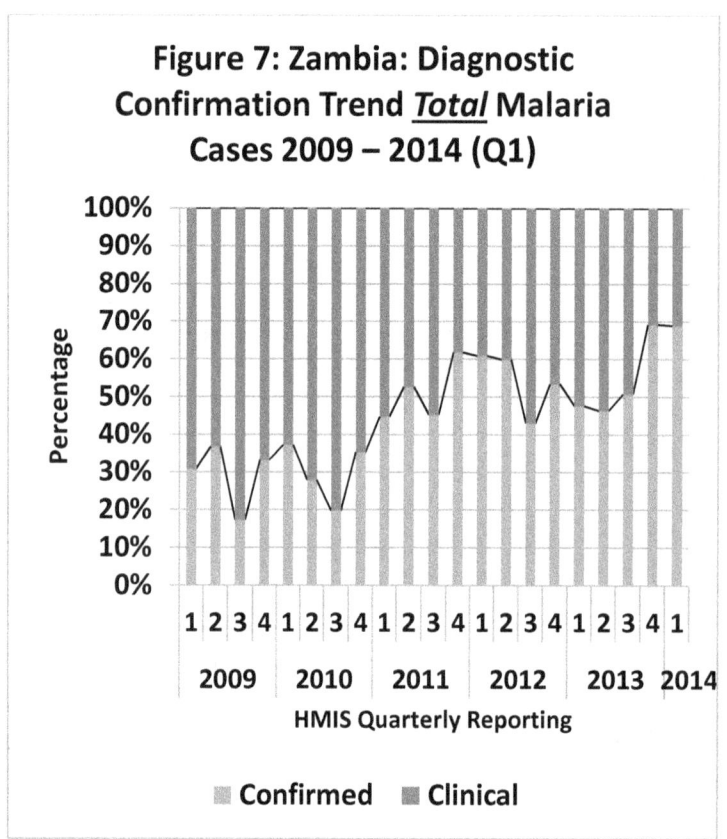

The RDT supply has improved. The PMI end-use verification survey (EUV) for the first quarter of FY 2014 reported no RDT stock outs in the health facilities visited. The quantification methodology for RDTs was adjusted for 2014. The need is now based on OPD attendance as reported in the HMIS, the estimated percent of OPD attendants with fever based on EUV reports, and then adjustments for community (additional 20%), inpatient requirements (30% of inpatient cases), and test & treat activities (600,000). This led to a significant increase in the estimated RDT need for Zambia in 2014 (18.7 million vs. 11.7 million).

In 2013, GRZ began procuring RDTs for the first time. A total of 10,756,000 RDTs arrived in Zambia in 2013 from procurements by GRZ (900,000), PMI (3,530,000 with FY 2012 funds), DFID (2,000,000 using PMI procurement mechanisms), and the Global Fund (4,326,000). In 2014, over 20,000,000 RDTs are expected to arrive with PMI providing 4,000,000 and DFID procuring 7.5 million.

To strengthen malaria diagnostic capacity at all levels, PMI has invested in training laboratory technicians, clinicians, and CHWs in malaria diagnosis—280 health facility workers and 439 CHWs in FY 2013. PMI supported the development and distribution of a laboratory training manual with standard operating procedures, the WHO accreditation of three laboratory technicians at the national level to build microscopy expertise and training capacity, and diagnostics refresher training for 18 district laboratory supervisors.

To ensure quality of malaria diagnostics, PMI supports the OTSS program. In OTSS, provincial and district-level supervisors visit health facilities using standardized checklists to observe microscopy and RDTs, recheck malaria smears, and collect information on provider adherence to laboratory results. These supervisors also provide on-site training and corrective action as needed. Through May 2014, 162 health facilities in all ten provinces participate in OTSS through 39 provincial and 30 district supervisors. PMI is also supporting the development of a comprehensive and sustainable national malaria diagnostics QA/QC framework.

Gap Analysis

Table J: Gap Analysis for RDTs 2014-2016			
	2014	**2015**	**2016**
RDT National Need	18,687,806	19,211,065	19,748,975
Three month pipeline	4,671,952		
Total Need	**23,359,758**	**19,211,065**	**19,748,975**
Commitments			
MOH	8,711,000	14,567,486	10,000,000
PMI	4,000,000	1,622,500	1,000,000
DFID	9,500,000	2,000,000	0
Malaria No More	600,000	0	0
Global Fund	4,100,000	3,211,065	3,500,000
Total Funded	**26,911,100**	**21,401,051**	**14,500,000**
Previous year surplus/gap	0	3,551,343	5,741,329
Annual RDT Surplus/Gap	**3,551,342**	**5,741,329**	**492,354**

Plans and justification

To provide health care workers, laboratory technicians, and CHWs with the tools to diagnose malaria, PMI will continue to support the procurement of malaria diagnostic commodities. PMI will procure 1,000,000 RDTs for use in health facilities and by CHWs. Also, reagents for microscopy will be provided for use by trained laboratory technicians at targeted facilities receiving OTSS.

PMI will continue to support roll out of OTSS to additional facilities as well as refresher training. The target number of facilities for full scale OTSS is 400, and by the end of 2014, 186 of the 400 will have participated in OTSS. Selection of health facilities for OTSS going forward will be based on diagnostic performance. High volume–low performance facilities will be targeted. PMI will also strengthen the quality of parasitological diagnosis in the public sector in four provinces through supportive supervision of healthcare providers at primary health facilities and community levels.

41

In addition, PMI will fund BCC activities focused on changing the expectations and practices of patients and caretakers.

Proposed activities with FY 2015 funding ($1,550,000)
- Procure 1,000,000 RDTs to be used at health facilities and by CHWs to contribute towards filling the RDT need in 2016, ($400,000);

- Strengthen malaria diagnostic capacity and quality assurance nationally through the training of malaria microscopists and support for OTSS. ($500,000);

- *Improve the quality of parasitological diagnosis in the public sector* in four targeted provinces through training and supportive supervision of healthcare providers at PHC and community levels. PMI will work at the provincial, district, and community level to improve the appropriate use of diagnostics including interpreting test results and managing patients based on results. This activity will begin during FY 2015 and expand to additional health facilities and the community with FY 2015 funding. ($600,000) ;

- Procure reagents and supplies to equip health centers for their malaria microscopy needs (417 health facilities have laboratories with microscopy), ($50,000);

- Support BCC activities to increase utilization and acceptance of diagnostics. (see BCC section)

Malaria Treatment

NMCP/PMI Objectives

All suspected malaria cases shall be subjected to parasite-based diagnosis and treatment initiated in accordance with the test result. The first-line drug for treatment of uncomplicated malaria in Zambia is artemether-lumefantrine (AL). A recent addition to the treatment guidelines is dihydroartemisin-piperaquine (DHA-PQ) as an alternative first-line choice for uncomplicated malaria. For uncomplicated malaria in pregnancy, the first-line treatments are: quinine in the first trimester and AL in the second and third trimesters.

The treatment of severe malaria has been updated in 2014. Injectable artesunate is the drug of choice in adults and children; if injectable (intravenous-IV or intramuscular-IM) artesunate is unavailable, artemether (IM) or quinine (IV or IM) are suggested alternatives. The new guidelines recommend that patients with severe malaria receive pre-referral treatment with IM or rectal artesunate; if that is not available, then IM quinine. The new guidelines state that the treatment of severe malaria in pregnancy is quinine in the first trimester and injectable artesunate in the second and third trimesters.

The MOH is supplementing volunteer CHWs with community health assistants (CHAs) in the hope of developing a sustainable, community-level cadre of health workers. CHAs are meant to be paid MOH employees and receive one year of training. A cadre of 307 CHAs was deployed in June 2012, and there was an additional cadre of 285 CHAs in 2013. CHAs are trained and equipped to diagnose and treat malaria, pneumonia, diarrhea and other illnesses (iCCM), and to spend 80% of their time in the community, and 20% of their time staffing health posts. They are to be supervised by the clinical team at health facilities. The goal is to train 1,114 CHAs by the end of 2015.

The volunteer CHW workforce has been active in Zambia since the 1970s providing preventive services and community mobilization. CHWs have an average of six weeks of formal training and use RDTs to diagnose malaria in children under-five years and treat positives with AL. CHWs in all districts in Luapula Province, and in three districts in each of the remaining provinces have been trained in the diagnosis and treatment of malaria, pneumonia and diarrhea (iCCM).

Zambia has a small private health sector that operates in larger towns and cities where the burden of malaria is lower than in rural areas. These providers have been informed of the use of AL as first-line treatment. Antimalarial drugs available in private pharmacies include AL, quinine, SP, and artemisinin monotherapies.

Progress during the last year

In 2014, the NMCP and partners made revisions to the Guidelines for the Diagnosis and Treatment of Malaria in Zambia that included: injectable artesunate for severe malaria, DHA-PQ as an alternate first-line treatment of uncomplicated malaria, and rectal artesunate for pre-referral treatment of severe malaria.

PMI procured 4,425,570 ACTs in 2014 for the treatment of malaria in health facilities and in the community. In addition, 4.3 million ACTs were procured with DFID funding, GRZ was planning to procure over 9 million, and Malaria No More purchased 1.6 million. If all procurements arrive in country as planned, Zambia will have full supply of ACTs for the first time.

The December 2013 EUV showed that 83% of malaria cases were treated with an ACT. This was an increase from 71% reported in September 2013. The MIS 2012 found that 85% of children under five that were given an antimalarial received an ACT.

PMI supports training and supervision of healthcare workers. In FY 2013, a total of 655 health workers in all provinces received training in malaria case management with ACTs which included the training of 439 CHWs in iCCM. An additional 159 CHWs have been trained in iCCM thus far in FY 2014. Supervision was supported via training of CCTs on supervisory skills specific to malaria case management. CCTs provide supervision for case management of malaria, with provincial level teams supervising district staffs, who in turn supervise staff at local health facilities. The OTSS program supported by PMI also works to improve adherence to test results and increase compliance with diagnostic and treatment algorithms for management of fever.

PMI partnered with the Clinton Health Access Initiative (CHAI) to begin the phased roll out of injectable artesunate for severe malaria. CHAI supported the trainings at one tertiary facility and five secondary facilities while PMI provided the artesunate commodity and technical assistance.

Once a facility is trained, the plan is to ensure adequate supply of artesunate. Thus the phased roll out is dependent on procurement of artesunate, and PMI at present is the only partner procuring.

AL maintains good efficacy in Zambia, as observed in a 2012 study conducted by the NMCP. The NMCP aims to do ACT efficacy studies regularly to ensure efficacy of first-line drugs. The PMI supported Drug Efficacy Study (DES) that was planned for the second quarter of FY 2014 has been delayed until first quarter FY 2015. This DES will include AL, ASAQ, and DHA-PQ. Another DES is planned for 2016 that will be funded through Global Fund.

Commodity gap analysis

The 2014 quantification exercise occurred in November 2013. Needs for ACTs are calculated based on "consumption" as reported by the 17 EMLIP districts and extrapolated to the rest of the country, and includes the need for a buffer stock to prevent stockouts. Injectable artesunate quantification was based on the number of inpatient cases in 2013 (135,814) disaggregated by age (<5 years 74,084; > 5 years 61,730). The under-fives would require one vial for a minimum of three doses, and the over-fives require is an estimated average of three vials for a minimum of three doses. A 10% decline of inpatient cases per year is anticipated.

Table K: Gap Analysis for ACTs 2013-2015 in Commodities Needed			
	2014	2015	2016
ACT National Need (# of treatments)	13,587,600	12,923,242	11,808,972
One month pipeline	1,132,300	1,076,937	984,081
Total Need	14,719,900	14,000,179	12,793,053
Commitments			
MOH	4,874,490	6,563,650	6,000,000
PMI	4,425,570	3,200,320	3,000,000
DFID	4,308,720	1,000,000	0
Malaria No More	1,599,920	500,000	0
Global Fund	0	3,133,242	2,808,972
Total Funded	15,208,700	14,397,212	11,808,972
Previous year surplus/gap	0	488,800	885,833
Annual ACT Surplus/Gap	488,800	885,833	(98,248)

Table L: Gap Analysis for Injectable Artesunate 2013-2015	2014	2015	2016
IAS National Need (# of 60mg vials)	777,822	700,040	630,036
One month pipeline	64,818	58,336	52,503
Total Need	842,640	758,376	682,539
Commitments			
MOH	0	0	0
PMI	20,000	120,000	120,000
Global Fund	0	0	0
Total Funded	20,000	120,000	120,000
Annual IAS Surplus/Gap	(822,640)	(638,376)	(562,539)

Plans and justification

The NMCP has prioritized technical support for case management as an area that PMI should address. The MIS 2012 indicated that among children under five with fever that received an anti-malarial drug, 85% reported receiving the recommended antimalarial (AL). This demonstrates tremendous progress from 2006 when only 18% received AL and 56% received SP. Thus, the priority going forward for PMI will be improving diagnostics, supportive supervision, roll out of injectable artesunate, and expanding access to treatment through iCCM.

With FY 2015 funding, PMI will work to increase prompt and effective treatment for uncomplicated malaria at the health facility level, expand access to injectable artesunate for severe malaria at hospital level, and support efforts to expand malaria treatment at the community level utilizing CHWs.

Proposed activities with FY 2015 funding ($4,500,000)
- Procure approximately 3,000,000 treatment courses of AL for uncomplicated malaria and 200,000 vials of artesunate 60mg for severe malaria. Semi-annual quantifications will monitor the supply and demand. ($3,300,000);

- Support the supervision of healthcare providers in the treatment of uncomplicated malaria and the training of CHWs in iCCM in four targeted provinces. Also, support the training of health workers at health facilities with inpatient services on the use of injectable artesunate for severe malaria. ($1,100,000);

- Support visits from the national level to monitor the quality of case management service delivery. ($100,000);

- Fund BCC messages and activities that focus on promoting use and adherence to recommended quality-assured ACTs. (see under BCC section)

Pharmaceutical Management

NMCP/PMI Objectives

The National Supply Chain Strategy for Essential Medicines (2013-2016) aims to provide equitable access to affordable, quality essential medicines and medical supplies to support the Zambian public health system. Key strategies of the MOH's strategic plan to achieve this objective include the following:

- Establish a coordinated and efficient supply chain in the sector led by one lead entity/point of reference.
- Reduce shortages of medical commodities and supplies within the supply chain by increasing the fill rate from the current 50% to 80%.
- Improve access to medical commodities and supplies though decentralizing distribution.
- Enhance accuracy in quantification and forecasting of medical commodities and supplies within the sector through provision of accurate data.
- Mobilize resources to support supply chain interventions in the sector
- Ensure sustained and improved quality for all medical commodities and supplies within the public health sector.
- Attain dynamic supply chain alignment and agility within the public health sector.
- Improve decision making processes through timely provision of information across the supply chain, by implementing appropriate supply chain information systems and technologies.
- Ensure private sector participation in the public health sector through various initiatives including Public Private Partnerships (PPPs).

During the strategic planning process, key supply chain objectives were grouped and defined into pillars that provide the framework around which the strategic objectives were formulated. These pillars are as follows:

- Quantification
- Procurement
- Logistics
- Information Systems
- Quality assurance and rational use
- Commodity security, financing and resource mobilization
- Performance management
- Human resources for health in supply chain
- Public Private Partnerships

In late 2012, the MOH announced the mandate of MSL would be significantly increased. In the past, MSL was responsible for central-level storage of commodities and distribution of those commodities to the district. Districts were then responsible for further distribution to health centers. The new policy expands MSL's mandate to include distribution to the health center. In order to expand its capacity for last mile distribution, MSL plans to create regional hubs and staging posts throughout the country. MSL's revised mandate also includes taking on roles that were previously the responsibility of the MOH's Procurement and Supply Unit. These roles include procurement, procurement planning, and quantification of essential medicines and medical supplies. The transfer of these activities is planned to be completed during 2014.

Progress during the last year

In 2014, MOH, with support from partners, redesigned the EMLIP to include health center kits. The combination of EMLIP and the kit are referred to as the EMLIP hybrid. Following improvements in essential medicines availability, in February 2014, the MOH officially adopted the hybrid system. In May 2014, the MOH allowed the rollout of the EMLIP hybrid system to resume. It is estimated that rollout of the EMLIP hybrid system will be completed by the end of 2016.

The Logistcs Management Unit at the MOH recorded a 98% reporting rate and improved commodity facility level stock availability (97%) for EMLIP districts for the period January to June 2014 of FY 2014. In addition, according to monthly reports sent to the LMU from health facilities, the percentage of health facilities stocked out of all presentations of ACT fell from 8% in June 2013 to 5% in April 2014.

With the re-initiation of EMLIP rollout, training for the EMLIP hybrid has been rolled out to nine new districts, which includes 294 health facilities and 588 health staff. This will bring the total coverage for EMLIP to 919 sites (target: 1,800 sites) and 2,402 health workers trained (target: 3,600 health workers).

PMI provided support to the MOH, MSL and other stakeholders to improve the collection, management, and use of logistics data through the development of an electronic Logistics Management Information System (eLMIS). In April 2014, the MOH approved the implementation of the eLMIS, an innovative tool which will electronically gather malaria logistics data (e.g., stock on hand, consumption, losses and adjustments) at facilities and transfers data electronically to MSL for order creation. eLMIS will replace the Supply Chain Manager. This will result in integration of logistics systems. Currently the eLMIS is being piloted at 48 sites in 8 selected districts. National rollout is planned for first quarter of FY 2015.

PMI continued to provide support to the national core group led by the MOH/NMCP to conduct annual and biannual forecasting and quantification exercises for ACTs, ITNs, RDTs, and SP. The national core group successfully conducted a transparent forecast and quantification exercise for 2014 through 2016. The entire process was facilitated by MOH/NMCP staff.

To improve strategic management and planning for increased commodity security, PMI provided support to the NMCP Malaria Case Management TWG. As part of this support, PMI contributed to the finalization of a costed National Supply Chain strategy (including an implementation plan). The final strategy is yet to be publicly released. Technical assistance was also provided in support of formulating a procurement strategy for MSL in view of its new mandates. Technical support was also provided to plan and implement a Community Health Assistance Logistics system.

Plans and justification

In collaboration with the MOH, PMI will continue strengthening the GRZ's commodities supply and logistics systems at central, provincial, district, and health center level. PMI will provide support for the continued rollout of EMLIP in collaboration with the MOH to improve the availability of malaria commodities at all levels of the health system. In addition, support will be provided to increase the MOH's ownership and coordination of forecasting, quantification and procurement planning for malaria commodities. PMI will continue to provide support to assess and monitor stock status for antimalarial drugs and RDTs at central, District Health Office, and health center levels. In support of MSL's new mandate, PMI will provide technical assistance to MSL to ensure successful adoption of its new tasks, including forecasting and supply planning capacity, as well as the improvement of the storage and distribution of malaria commodities.

Proposed activities with FY 2015 funding ($1,032,900)

Assist the MOH in the roll out of EMLIP hybrid as well as provide technical assistance to strengthen pharmaceutical and supply chain management systems. Specific activities will include the following:

- Provide technical assistance for quarterly forecasting of antimalarial drug and RDT needs and gaps in all districts ($100,000);

- Importing, quality control, storage, distribution, and inventory management down to the health facility level (included in commodity procurement line items);

- Provide technical assistance to support the rollout of EMLIP including training health workers and improving feedback and reporting on consumption/stocks from health facility to district and higher levels ($575,000);

- Monitoring of implementation/evaluation of coverage ($57,900);

- End-use verification/monitoring of availability of key antimalarial commodities at the facility level in a sample of all districts. Specifically, EUV entails the regular supervisory/monitoring visits to a sampling of health facilities to detect: ACT (or other drug) stock outs; expiration dates of ACTs at health facilities; leakage; anomalies in ACT use by clinicians; and to verify quantification/consumption assumptions; and ($100,000)

- Provide technical assistance to MSL in support of its new mandate. ($200,000)

5.   Behavior Change Communication

NMCP/PMI Objectives

The NMCP's BCC strategy for 2011–2014 has clear behavior change objectives for each of the malaria control interventions, and also identifies barriers to the desired behaviors as well as problem behaviors that compete with the desired behaviors. Target audiences are also identified and measurable communication objectives are clearly stipulated. Finally, for each control intervention, messages are articulated and a media mix suggested. All institutions working on malaria in the public, private, non-governmental organizations (NGOs), and PMI partners are to follow the national strategy.

Progress during the last year

The recently released 2012 MIS included several knowledge-based indicators linked to BCC that indicate high knowledge of appropriate preventive and curative measures for malaria, in women 15–49 years of age (Table J). Although knowledge is not equivalent to "practice" nor is it a guarantee that an individual will exhibit the target behavior to prevent or treat malaria, it does indicate to a certain extent that BCC activities in Zambia have been successful at increasing and maintaining awareness about malaria.

Table M: General malaria knowledge among women ages 15 – 49 years (2006 -2012)		
Indicator	**2006**	**2012**
Percentage who had heard of malaria	96	96
Percentage who recognized fever as a symptom of malaria	64	78
Percentage who reported mosquito bites as a cause of malaria	77	89
Percentage who reported mosquito nets as a prevention method	76	86

Source: Zambia National Malaria Indicator Survey 2012. National Malaria Control Program. May 2013. N=2,699.

When queried about the sources of information in the 2012 MIS, women aged 15–49 who had heard about malaria (96%), 67% had heard a message from a health provider and 42% had heard it from other sources (including PMI-supported BCC); there was some overlap on sources of information, as expected. Surprisingly, malaria messages of one sort or another are prevalent in the BCC target group as the average number of months since last hearing a malaria message was three months. Although urban dwellers fared a little better in their knowledge about malaria, knowledge was very similar across provinces, wealth indices, and levels of education, attesting to the wide dissemination of malaria messages.

As suggested by the national BCC strategy, PMI supports several vehicles for its communication activities. A PMI partner has been implementing an integrated community-based communications initiative called "Champion Communities" focusing on promotion of malaria prevention, diagnosis, appropriate treatment, and nutrition for pregnant women and children under five in 8 districts and 131 communities across four higher malaria burden provinces since 2011. The Champion Communities initiative is a facilitated, participatory methodology to motivate communities to set and work towards goals. In this initiative, communities establish their own goals and action plans, design their own community activities, conduct monthly self-monitoring, and use public presentation of the data/progress towards goals to motivate everyone in the community to participate. A cadre of community malaria agents meets monthly with each participating household to provide counseling as well as to collect data on key behaviors. These data points are then aggregated and presented back to each community for discussion and processing. The objectives of the initiative are:

- Increase the number of children under five and pregnant women who sleep under an ITN every night.
- Increase number of pregnant women who attend antenatal care early and receive three recommended doses of IPTp.
- Increase number of pregnant women and children under five who go for immediate malaria testing and treatment at first symptoms.
- Increase number of caregivers who appropriately feed children suffering from malaria.
- It involves monthly mini household surveys combined with on-the-spot counseling on issues that arise. The communities also hold monthly community meetings to discuss aggregate results from surveys and progress towards goals.

By August 2013, the initiative had recorded impressive results, with the proportion of pregnant women who attended antenatal care increasing from 60% to 93% and the proportion of eligible pregnant women who received IPTp increasing from 55% to 95% in the targeted communities. The proportion of persons who had a fever in the past two weeks who got a malaria test increased from 70% to 87% while the proportion of persons who slept under an ITN increased from 48%to 65%. This successful approach will continue to be utilized in similar activities in targeted districts in the future.

As Zambia advances in its control of malaria in the Southern Province and beyond, the behavioral issues it will encounter will be more and more complex and likely demand further investment to resolve them. Improving coverage of some interventions will likely slow down as early adopters of malaria interventions have already been reached while late adopters require additional and innovative convincing to adopt and maintain behaviors that, up to now, they have rejected. Late adopters may not be homogenously distributed in the population and it will require special efforts to identify and reach them.

Plans and justification

All PMI indicators have human behavior components. They are dependent on the presence of the appropriate commodity and the right incentives and motivation of individuals to use those commodities. A mix of communication activities—mass media, community, and interpersonal— is necessary to inform, promote, and maintain the behaviors to prevent and treat malaria. The mix of activities is dependent on the types of behaviors, barriers to behaviors, and whether the behavior has reached a critical mass in the population. However, in all cases, communication activities need to be sustained or the behavior will change over time, as the risk is perceived to have disappeared.

Proposed activities with FY 2015 funding ($2,200,000)

The NMCP believes that both national and community BCC activities are needed to change and maintain behaviors in malaria prevention and treatment. Each approach reaches different audiences and reinforces key messages. The final mix of mass, community, and interpersonal communication activities; technical orientation; and geographic locale will be based on evidence that will help focus efforts. A part of the M&E strategy for BCC will be through the regular MIS that collects knowledge and practice information as well coverage estimates (final results of

BCC efforts). Emphasis will be to maintain current levels of coverage and expand to cohorts that have been difficult to reach or are recalcitrant in adopting the desired behaviors. The list below provides potential tasks and their rationale.

- National BCC to maintain ownership and proper use of ITNs through national multi-media efforts. Net use lags behind ownership, and needs both community and national efforts to achieve an increase. National activities will focus on at least three groups; first, maintenance of appropriate behaviors in the population that is already exhibiting them; second, introduction of new cohorts to the desired behaviors; and, third reaching late adopters and those that are difficult to reach geographically ($180,000);

- Community-based BCC in four targeted provinces through NGOs/Faith-based organizations to increase net ownership and use. Zambia has good ITN ownership and use indicators in the general population, but late adopters require a more focused and interpersonal approach ($550,000);

- National BCC to increase ANC attendance and demand for IPTp. Every year, there is a new cohort of primigravid women. Therefore, continued investment is required for outreach activities related to malaria in pregnancy. National BCC efforts for malaria in pregnancy are part of a larger integrated campaign on maternal health and nutrition that disseminates messages through national radio and television spots ($100,000);

- Community-based BCC in four targeted provinces to increase ANC attendance and demand for IPTp. BCC activities through community groups (SMAGs) will be implemented to increase use of IPTp ($540,000);

- National BCC campaign to increase ACT usage. Care seeking outside the home is relatively high in Zambia. Still, not all patients seek treatment at a health facility. Mass media activities will promote early care seeking and treatment of malaria cases in children under five years of age ($80,000); and

- Community-based BCC campaign in four targeted provinces through NGOs/faith-based organizations (FBOs) to increase ACT usage. This activity has the same objectives as the national BCC campaign but its focus is on community-level activities support by NGOs/FBOs ($550,000).

- Support to rollout national BCC strategy ($200,000)

6.   Monitoring and Evaluation

NMCP/PMI Objectives

The revised Zambia NMSP 2011-2016 states the objective of Surveillance, Monitoring & Evaluation is to: "strengthen surveillance, M&E systems in order to ensure timely availability of quality, consistent and relevant data on malaria control performance by 2016." This data is to guide policy and decision-making. Along with the revised NMSP, a revised National M&E Plan will be developed to address the challenges in Zambia as it moves along malaria's epidemiological continuum. The M&E strategy tracks all Roll Back Malaria-recommended indicators. Three M&E strategies are:

1. Strengthen coordination/ collaboration in surveillance, monitoring and evaluation
2. Data management systems—strengthen the implementation of data management systems at community, facility, district, provincial and national levels to efficiently collect, process, analyze, and manage malaria transmission and disease data
3. Surveillance to track progress towards elimination—strengthen capacities of health personnel at all levels with the aim of improving quality and timeliness of case detection and reporting

PMI's support to M&E in Zambia aligns with the NMSP and the National Malaria M&E Plan. PMI coordinates and collaborates with the NMCP and several partners in providing technical assistance and resources for M&E activities including MACEPA, the Global Fund, UNICEF, and WHO.

Monitoring: Malaria cases are reported through the National HMIS using a combination of paper tools and the DHIS2. All public and mission health facilities and some private facilities are to report health data monthly through the HMIS. Information flows from the health facility to the district and provincial level before being transmitted to the HMIS group within the MOH. The NMCP accesses malaria data from the MOH HMIS and maintains its own web-based data management system using the DHIS2 platform. The HMIS collects data on malaria clinical and confirmed cases, OPD and inpatient cases, and deaths by age under 1 year, 1–5 years, and over five years.

Evaluation: To evaluate outcomes and impact of malaria prevention and control activities in Zambia, nationally-representative surveys such as the DHS and the MIS are performed periodically. All-cause mortality in children under five years of age is tracked using the DHS; other child health indicators are also collected by the DHS and used in assessing impact. The last DHS report is from 2007 and provides a baseline estimate of mortality at the start of PMI. Data collection for the 2014 DHS has been completed with a preliminary report expected by the end of the year.

A nationwide MIS was carried out in 2006, 2008, 2010, and 2012 to provide information on the coverage of the four major malaria interventions, malaria parasite prevalence, and the prevalence of severe anemia, and is useful for measuring changes over time. The next MIS will occur in 2015.

A number of other non-PMI-financed surveys and evaluations provide additional provincial-, district-, and community-level data on malaria epidemiology in Zambia, and provide useful information on the progress of malaria control efforts. These include health facility surveys to assess health worker performance and the quality of health care, availability of health guidelines, personnel, and equipment, and household surveys to assess knowledge, attitudes, and practices related to malaria. As part of routine supervisory visits to MOH facilities, checklists are also completed on health worker performance and other technical aspects of health care. Table N shows household and facility surveys implemented and planned from 2004 to 2016.

Table N: Surveillance, Monitoring and Evaluation Data Sources, 2004 – 2016

Data Sources	2004	2005	2006	2007	2008	2009	2010	2011	2012	2013	2014	2015	2016
Household surveys													
DHS				X							X		
MIS			X*		X		X		X			(X)	
Roll Back Malaria Baseline	X*												
Knowledge, Attitudes and Practices Survey						X*							
Health Facility and Other Surveys													
IMCI Health Facility Survey					X*								
WHO Service Availability Mapping			X*										
Health Facility Survey	X*	X*						X					(X)
End-Use Verification						X	X	X	X	X	X		
Electronic Logistics Management Information System (eLMIS)											X	(X)	
Malaria Surveillance and Routine Systems													
HMIS/DHIS2										X*	X*	(X)	
Malaria Surveillance (Rapid reporting)													
Therapeutic Efficacy Monitoring													
In-vivo therapeutic efficacy									X	X	X	(X)	
Entomological surveillance													
Entomological surveillance and resistance monitoring								X*	X	X	X	(X)	
Other data sources													
Malaria Program							X			X			

Review					
Progress in child health across districts in Zambia (MCEP, IHME)		X*			
MalariaCare		X	X	X	(X)	(X)
IRS (AIRS)		X	X	X	(X)	(X)

* Not financed by PMI
() Planned activity

Progress during the last year

<u>Mid-Term Review:</u> The Zambia Mid-Term Review (MTR) of the NMSP 2011-2015 was completed in October 2013. The MTR was conducted under the leadership and coordination of the MOH Directorate of Disease Control Surveillance & Research, with support from malaria control partners and stakeholders. The MTR assessed the progress made against the goals, objectives, and targets outlined in the plan, identified the key challenges hindering progress, and recommend improvements for performance to assure impact in the remaining period of the NMSP 2011-2015. The report provided direction for revising the NMSP and extending the plan through 2016.

Key Findings and Recommendations from the MTR:
- The epidemiology of malaria in Zambia is diverse with areas of high transmission to areas of little or no malaria. Understanding the local epidemiology is increasingly important to maximize malaria control resources.
- It is critical that technical working groups have regularly scheduled meetings to make progress in implementing a coordinated malaria control and elimination agenda.
- Malaria control and elimination work is increasingly borne by districts. It is recommended to advocate for malaria focal point persons and a malaria surveillance officer at the district level to help coordinate district malaria control and surveillance efforts.
- The NMCP should continue to strategically use IRS to mitigate insecticide resistance and maximize malaria burden reduction, complementing current universal ITN efforts.
- As the program pursues malaria elimination in some areas, greater attention should be given to Surveillance Monitoring and Evaluation, and Operational Research and BCC. Furthermore, care must be taken not to prematurely withdraw prevention activities from the malaria free areas.
- It is further recommended to continue to develop new strategies that will effectively reduce malaria where current strategies, despite successful implementation, have not yielded optimal results.

<u>HMIS:</u> The national HMIS has been upgraded from the District Health Information System (DHIS) 1.4 to 2.0, offering significant improvements in timeliness of reporting, data visualization and data systems management. DHIS2 has now been rolled out to all districts in the country. Capacity building activities have been conducted at all levels of the health system in

surveillance, monitoring, and evaluation. WHO reports that in 2013 the reporting rate for health facilities was 90%—20,124 reports out of 22,308 expected (1,859 facilities x 12 months). Using the DHIS2 System, data may be analyzed using maps, charts, pivot tables, or summarized through dashboards. Malaria data from the HMIS is being used to follow trends in incidence at the district level, targeting health facility catchment areas for IRS, locating hot spots in very low endemic areas, and following trends in confirmed cases and diagnostic use.

Figure 8: District examples from the DHIS2

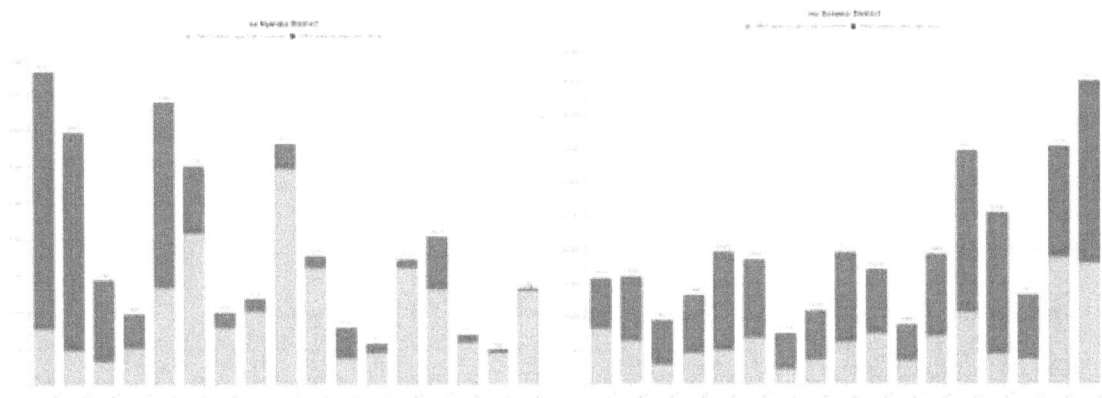

Rapid Reporting: Malaria surveillance systems were developed for Southern Province at the facility level using the malaria rapid reporting system, mobile phones, and geographic information system. Health care workers report malaria cases, lab testing, and drug availability by web-enabled cell phones on a weekly basis. This data can be accessed through DHIS2 online platform. This rapid reporting system has been expanded to additional facilities in Western and Central Provinces.

Active Infection Detection: The previously PMI-supported enhanced surveillance in Lusaka District has been transitioned over to the Lusaka District Health Office. Active Infection Detection is ongoing in 23 of the 28 district health facilities. PMI support has shifted to Mumbwa District where Active Infection Detection has begun. Community-level malaria reactive case detection continues in very low prevalence areas in Southern Province.

End-Use Verification: The EUV collects data on malaria commodities every month from facilities to assess availability. The last report for EUV is for the first quarter of 2014. The data reported is from districts in which EMLIP has been rolled out. Eleven EMLIP health facilities were visited. No facilities were stocked out of all ACTs and consequently would not be able to treat malaria cases. The facilities had varying degrees (18%–50%) of stock outs of the different ACTs. The index of ACT availability shown in Figure 9 shows a small improvement from 1st quarter 2013. The 2014 EUV reports only one facility with an RDT stock out.

Figure 9: Index of AL availability in health facilities, EUV, 1st Quarter 2013 (23 facilities) and 2014 (11 facilities)

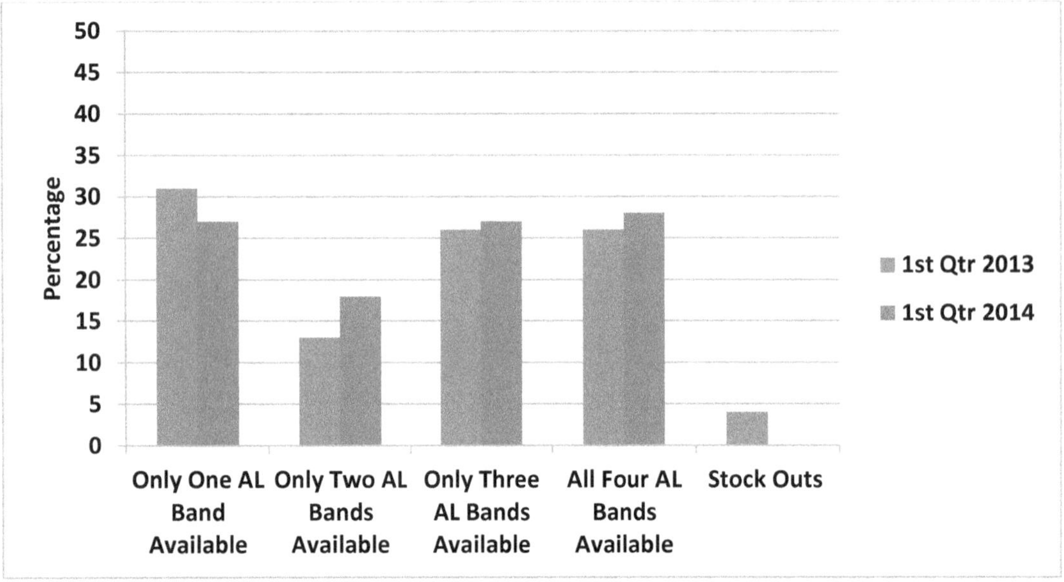

Note: each band is a dose packet size.
Source: End Use Verification report, 1ˢᵗ Quarter 2013 and 2014

<u>Field Epidemiology Training Program (FETP)</u>: CDC reached agreements with the MOH, MCDMCH, and the University of Zambia to begin the FETP in Zambia. Six FETP residents will start in August 2014. One PMI-supported malaria resident will be posted at the MOH/NMCC.

Plans and justification

Monitoring and evaluating malaria control activities will rely on a combination of routine malaria data through the HMIS and surveys. With FY 2015 funds, PMI will provide support to strengthen routine malaria data collection at the health facility, district, and provincial levels through the HMIS. The objective is to achieve 100% on-time reporting of malaria cases by districts and 90% by health facilities in PMI-targeted provinces. PMI will also support a health facility survey and two FETP residents. With FY 2015 funds, PMI intends to support the following activities:

Proposed activities with FY 2015 funding ($1,173,400)

- Strengthen routine M&E systems (HMIS) in four targeted provinces. PMI will help strengthen the HMIS at health facility, district, and provincial levels. Implementation activities will include: support for training and supervision of data clerical staff at health facilities and district community health offices including support to DHIS2; improving collection and reporting of routine malaria indicators at community level; and strengthening malaria data analysis and use for planning and decision making ($400,000);

- Support a health facility survey in 2016. This survey will be implemented five years after the last one (2011) and will provide follow-up of data on performance of the malaria program at the facility level, including: case management skills, interpersonal communication, availability of malaria commodities, management of pre-referrals, etc. ($300,000);

- Provide resources for central-level NMCP personnel to conduct and follow up on data quality audits in all districts and provincial offices in one year. This activity entails visiting officers responsible for collecting, collating, and reporting data from health facilities to higher levels of the health system and ensuring that appropriate quality procedures are followed. No other donors are currently funding this activity ($100,000);

- Monitor attrition/survivorship and physical integrity of ITNs following mass campaign ($100,000);

- CDC technical assistance for routine monitoring of net durability ($12,100);

- CDC technical assistance in monitoring and evaluation activities ($12,100);

- Support training of two NMCP and/or provincial-level staff in epidemiologic methods, data analysis techniques, operations research, and strategic information for public health decision making through Zambia FETP ($150,000).

7. Operational Research (OR)

Completed OR studies
A PMI-funded study of the efficacy of sulfadoxine-pyrimethamine for IPTpin Mansa, Zambia was completed in 2013. (see the MIP section for more information.)

Ongoing OR studies
PMI supported an operational research project on ITN durability that is currently ongoing (see ITN section). This study examining structural integrity of ITNs distributed in Northern and Luapula Provinces was started in 2011 and has since finished field work at the end of 2013. Preliminary results indicate significant deterioration by 12 months of age, with 66% attrition by 30 months of age, suggesting a more abbreviated lifespan of ITNs than previously believed. Baseline results of the study were presented at an ASTMH conference in 2013, and preliminary results have been presented to the MOH/NMCC. Pending results on insecticide content of the ITNs via bioassays and chemical analysis, final analysis and a manuscript is anticipated for late 2014.

Planned OR studies
A recent policy change in Zambia now emphasizes universal coverage of LLINs with focal or targeted IRS. Historically, vector control was split, with IRS reserved for urban and peri-urban areas while LLINs were targeted to rural areas. This approach in vector control has been ineffective, leading to increases in malaria cases in several districts throughout the country.

The new approach to vector control may be more cost-effective and ultimately could have a greater impact on malaria control and prevention in Zambia. Unfortunately, little data exists to help drive the decision-making process of determining where IRS would be best targeted in combination with universal LLIN coverage. The OR study proposed would help shed light on this issue in Zambia. It will also contribute to the limited scientific body of knowledge regarding the added benefit of IRS in combination with LLINs.

Given the recent progress Zambia has made progress in malaria case management, NMCP has looked to new approaches to further this progress. The use of rectal artesunate as pre-referral treatment was added to NMCP policy in 2014. At the time of MOP writing, this policy is not being implemented and commodities have not been secured. It has yet to be determined in which areas in Zambia that pre-referral treatment with rectal artesunate would be more effective and what criteria should be used to make this determination. The robustness of the referral network is an important aspect to understand in selecting where this new approach to pre-referral treatment should be added to the current case management arsenal. The proposed OR study would provide more information about the robustness of the referral network in selected areas as the first step in understanding the best use of rectal artesunate for pre-referral treatment.

Table O: Summary of Operations Research			
Completed OR Studies			
Title	Start Date	End Date	Budget
The efficacy of SP for IPTp, Mansa, Zambia	January 2010	Published June 2014	$200,000
Ongoing OR Studies			
Title	Start Date	End Date	Budget
ITN prospective study	2011		$50,000
Planned OR Studies			
Title	Start Date	End Date	Budget
Focal IRS with LLINs study	2014 (pending approval)		$400,000
Assessment of referral network for severe malaria	2014 (pending approval)		$75,000

Proposed activities with FY 2015 funding ($24,200)

- PMI is supporting operations research in Zambia that will help clarify several important issues. CDC will provide two technical assistance visits to support the on-going OR ($24,200);

8. Health System Strengthening and Capacity Building

NMCP/PMI Objectives

As mentioned previously, the public health sector in Zambia has been re-organized. There are now two ministries sharing responsibilities for the health portfolio. The MOH is tasked with service delivery at levels 2 and 3 health facilities, surveillance, monitoring and evaluation, resource mobilization, and research. The MCDMCH is tasked with service delivery at district and community level including, FANC and malaria case management from the district level to the local level. The NMCP has staff from both the MOH and the MCDMCH. Plans for co-locating staff from the two ministries at the NMCC are at an advanced stage. The malaria unit at the MCDMCH is under the Directorate of Maternal and Child Health and currently has three staff positions; Malaria Specialist, Malaria Epidemiologist and Integrated Vector Control Officer. The NMCC is a department under the Directorate of Disease Surveillance, Control and Research of the MOH, and provides technical oversight to malaria activities in public health facilities to the provincial level, as well as supporting and coordinating a wide range of partners, including research and training institutions. The NMCP has 10 staff positions, including a Case Management Officer, Chief Entomologist, Chief Parasitologist, Malaria Epidemiologist, BCC, IRS, Surveillance and Information, an ITN Officer, a Medical Laboratory Technologist, and an OR Officer. At the provincial level, Provincial Health Offices serve as an extension of the MOH, while the DCMOs serve as extensions of the MCDMCH and have the fiscal authority to manage district health centers and health posts and therefore become the main implementers of the IRS program.

The NMCP staff is committed to scaling-up malaria control and prevention activities; however, they are currently understaffed, and need further support to effectively supervise provincial- and district-level activities and effectively coordinate the many partners contributing to malaria efforts in Zambia. In particular, the NMCP and partners recognize its need for additional coordination of malaria commodity procurement and supply chain management, IRS activities, and advocacy and outreach efforts. The NMCP requires support to conduct provincial-level visits for supervision and program management which MACEPA and PMI are providing. PMI will continue to provide support for IRS training, mapping of households, entomology expertise, and assistance for NMCP in gathering and analysis of malaria data.

Progress during the last year

The PMI Zambia team has been providing technical assistance and capacity building at the NMCP, including M&E. Time spent at NMCP by PMI RAs will continue as a priority. The PMI Zambia team will continue to work closely with the NMCC and the Malaria Epidemiologist at the MCDMCH malaria unit to help build their capacity in M&E.

USAID partners for BCC, health systems strengthening, and social marketing activities have formed close partnerships with civil society organizations, including NGOs, community-based organizations, and faith-based groups in order to scale up the delivery of high-quality malaria prevention and treatment interventions. To enhance national capacity in this area, the PMI BCC partner will support the NMCP in their national campaigns including campaigns on ITNs and IRS.

In FY 2014 DFID took up funding of the National Professional Officer for malaria position at the Zambia WHO Country Office that was previously funded by PMI. DFID committed to fund the position through FY 2015, with funding channeled through USAID. The National Professional Officer provided technical leadership for the mid-term review of the NMSP 2011-2016. He also provided technical support towards development of the Global Fund Application for malaria, planning for the mass ITN country-wide campaign aimed at achieving universal coverage, and for the revision of 2010 national malaria treatment guidelines.

An opportunity for NMCP capacity building is the initiation of CDC's FETP program in Zambia in August 2014, with a second cohort starting a year later. The FETP program is a two-year applied epidemiology training program that results in a Master of Science degree. PMI will support one candidate per year, alternating assignment between the MOH/NMCC and MCDMCH ministries. The program is open only to Zambian nationals.

Proposed activities with FY 2014 funding ($60,000)

- Provide funds through a government-to-government mechanism for NMCP staff travel and training. This will support NMCP staff to attend meetings such as the American Society for Tropical Medicine and Hygiene, regional M&E, or commodity quantification workshops, ($60,000);

- Support for two Zambian nationals to participate in a FETP program. This activity will support long-term local capacity within the MOH, (see under M&E section).

9.   Staffing and Administration

Two health professionals serve as Resident Advisors (RAs) to oversee the PMI in Zambia, one representing CDC and one representing USAID. In addition, one or more Foreign Service Nationals work as part of the PMI team. All PMI staff members are part of a single inter-agency team led by the USAID Mission Director or his/her designee in country. The PMI team shares responsibility for development and implementation of PMI strategies and work plans, coordination with national authorities, managing collaborating agencies, and supervising day-to-day activities. Candidates for RA positions (whether initial hires or replacements) will be evaluated and/or interviewed jointly by USAID and CDC, and both agencies will be involved in hiring decisions, with the final decision made by the individual agency.
The PMI professional staff work together to oversee all technical and administrative aspects of the PMI, including finalizing details of the project design, implementing malaria prevention and treatment activities, monitoring and evaluation of outcomes and impact, reporting of results, and providing guidance to PMI partners.

The PMI lead in-country is the USAID Mission Director. The two PMI RAs, one from USAID and one from CDC, report to the Senior USAID Health Officer for day-to-day leadership, and work together as a part of a single interagency team. The technical expertise housed in Atlanta and Washington guides PMI programmatic efforts and thus overall technical guidance for both RAs falls to the PMI staff in Atlanta and Washington. Since CDC resident advisors are CDC employees (CDC USDD—38), responsibility for completing official performance reviews lies with the CDC Country Director who is expected to rely upon input from PMI staff across the two agencies that work closely day in and day out with the CDC RA and thus best positioned to comment on the RA's performance.

The two PMI RAs are based within the USAID Health Office and are expected to spend approximately half their time sitting with and providing technical assistance to the national malaria control programs and partners.

Locally-hired staff to support PMI activities either in Ministries or in USAID will be approved by the USAID Mission Director. Because of the need to adhere to specific country policies and USAID accounting regulations, any transfer of PMI funds directly to Ministries or host governments will need to be approved by the USAID Mission Director and Controller, in addition to the USG Global Malaria Coordinator.

Table 1
President's Malaria Initiative – Zambia
(FY 2015) Budget Breakdown by Partner

Partner	Geographical Area	Activity	Budget ($)	%
TBD (Procurement and Supply Chain)	National	Procurement of ACTs, RDTs, lab supplies, roll out of logistics system.	$8,182,900	34.1%
MalariaCare	National	Strengthen malaria diagnostic capacity and quality assurance nationally through the training of malaria microscopists and support for OTSS.	$500,000	2.1%
TBD (IRS)	40 districts (29 original districts)	Procurement of insecticides for IRS. Support environmental monitoring, insecticide resistance monitoring	$8,144,500	33.9%
TBD (Bilateral Project)	National and 4 Provinces	Improve the quality of parasitological diagnosis in the public sector in four provinces; strengthen FANC in four targeted provinces, community-based BCC, roll out additional continuous LLIN distribution channels in selected provinces/districts, technical assistance to strengthen HMIS.	$4,590,000	19.1%
TBD (BCC)	National	Support to national-level BCC activities.	$560,000	2.3%
PeaceCorps	District	Support OR	$10,000	0.04%
CDC-IAA	NA	Entomologic monitoring and insecticide resistance, M&E, net durability, operations research and FETP training	$222,600	0.9%
USAID-CDC Staff	NA	Personnel	$1,230,000	5.1%
NMCP	NA	District and provincial data audits, M&E, support for health facility survey	$560,000	2.3%
Total			**$24,000,000**	**100%**

Table 2
President's Malaria Initiative – Zambia
Planned Obligations for Year 7 (FY 2014) ($24,000,000)

Proposed Activity	Mechanism	Budget Total $	Budget Commodity $	Geographical area	Description
PREVENTIVE ACTIVITIES					
Insecticide Treated Nets					
Procurement of LLINs	TBD	3,000,000	3,000,000	National	Procure LLINs for routine/continuous distribution.
LLIN Distribution	TBD	400,000		National	Support the storage and distribution of LLINs, including transportation and other logistics, to districts and health facilities.
Provide technical assistance to roll out innovative, effective strategies for sustaining high LLIN coverage	TBD	300,000		TBD	Roll out additional continuous LLIN distribution channels in selected provinces/districts
SUBTOTAL ITNs		**3,700,000**	**3,000,000**		
Indoor Residual Spraying					
Procurement of IRS commodities and support to other components of the program.	TBD	6,170,500	6,170,500	40 districts (29 original districts)	Procure insecticides and other IRS supplies/equipment for spraying up to 450,000 structures. Support environmental monitoring and environmental assessment
Implementation of IRS program, monitoring and evaluation, storage/incinerator, community sensitization, geocoding, BCC	TBD	1,674,000		40 districts (29 original districts)	Training, monitoring and evaluation, and BCC for IRS; pesticide storage, waste disposal.
Entomological monitoring and insecticide resistance monitoring and support to insectary	TBD	300,000		NA	Support insectary and entomological monitoring
CDC technical assistance on entomological monitoring and insecticide resistance	CDC IAA	24,200		NA	Provide technical assistance on entomological monitoring and insecticide resistance.

Activity	Funder	Budget	Budget	Location	Description
SUBTOTAL IRS		8,168,700	6,170,500		
Intermittent Preventive Treatment in Pregnancy					
Strengthening of FANC for IPTp	TBD	450,000		National and 4 provinces	Strengthen FANC in four targeted provinces.
SUBTOTAL IPTp		450,000	0		
SUBTOTAL PREVENTIVE		12,318,700	9,170,500		
Case Management					
Diagnosis					
Procure rapid diagnostic tests	TBD	400,000	400,000	National	Procure RDTs for health facilities and iCCM
Strengthen malaria diagnostic capabilities at the health center level	MalariaCare	500,000		National	Strengthen malaria diagnostic capacity and quality assurance nationally through the training of malaria microscopists and support for OTSS.
Improve the quality of parasitological diagnosis in the public sector in four provinces	TBD	600,000		National and 4 targeted provinces	Training and supportive supervision of healthcare providers at PHC and community levels to improve the appropriate use of diagnostics
Procure reagents and supplies	TBD	50,000	50,000	National	Procure reagents and supplies for microscopy
SUBTOTAL – Diagnosis		1,550,000	450,000		
Treatment & Pharmaceutical Management					
Procure ACTs	TBD	3,300,000	3,300,000	National	Procure ACTs for the treatment of malaria in facilities and communities and procure injectable artesunate to support the roll-out of injectable artesunate in line with updated national malaria case management guidelines
Strengthen facility- and community-based treatment with ACTs	TBD	1,100,000		National	Training, supervision support, to improve service delivery in health facilities including treatment of malaria, and to assist with roll-out into communities through CHWs. Train health workers in new guidelines

Activity	Detailed description	Location	Cost (US$)		Funding source
Supervisory visits from central level	Supervisory visits from central level to provincial health facilities to review malaria case management.	National	100,000		NMCP
Roll out the national logistics and pharmaceutical management system for malaria commodities	Strengthen supply chain and logistics for all malaria commodities and essential drugs, including Pharmaceutical Regulatory Authority and the End Use Tool	National	1,032,900		TBD
SUBTOTAL – Treatment & Pharmaceutical Management			**5,532,900**	**3,300,000**	
SUBTOTAL CASE MANAGEMENT			**7,082,900**	**3,750,000**	
BCC					
National BCC to maintain ownership and proper use of ITNs through national multimedia efforts	BCC for net usage at national level	National	180,000		TBD
Community-based BCC through NGOs/FBOs to increase net ownership and use	BCC for net usage at community level in four targeted provinces	Four targeted provinces	550,000		TBD
National BCC to increase ANC attendance and demand for IPTp	BCC for IPTp promotion at national level	National	100,000		TBD
Community-based BCC to increase ANC attendance and demand for IPTp	BCC for IPTp at community level in four targeted provinces	Four targeted provinces	540,000		TBD
National BCC campaign to increase ACT usage	BCC for promotion of care seeking and ACT usage at national level	National	80,000		TBD
Community-based BCC campaign through NGOs/FBOs to increase ACT usage	BCC for community-level care seeking and ACT usage in four targeted provinces	Four targeted provinces	550,000		TBD
Support to rollout national BCC strategy	Support to rollout national BCC strategy	National	200,000		TBD
SUBTOTAL BCC			**2,200,000**		
Monitoring and Evaluation/Operations Research					
Support for a health facility survey	Support health facility survey	National	300,000		NMCP
Technical assistance to strengthen HMIS	Technical assistance to strengthen HMIS in four targeted provinces	Four targeted provinces	400,000		TBD
District and provincial data audits	Resources for central level personnel to conduct and follow up data quality audits in all districts and provincial offices in one year	NMCP	100,000		NMCP
Technical assistance for M&E	Technical assistance on monitoring and evaluation issues.	NA	12,100		CDC-IAA

Description	Funder	Amount		Notes
Routine monitoring of net durability	TBD	100,000	TBD	Routine monitoring of net durability
Technical assistance for routine monitoring of net durability	CDC-IAA	12,100		Technical assistance for routine monitoring of net durability
Field Epidemiology Training Program	CDC-IAA	150,000	National	Training for two Zambian nationals in field epidemiology
Technical assistance for OR	CDC-IAA	24,200	NA	Technical assistance on operations research
SUBTOTAL - M & E		**1,098,400**	**0**	
Health System Strengthening and Capacity Building				
Training and travel to build capacity of NMCP staff	NMCP	60,000	National	Fund travel and registration to international meetings such as MIM, SARN, and ASTMH and regional trainings. Support strategy development.
SUBTOTAL Capacity Bldg.		**60,000**	**0**	
In-country Staffing and Administration				
In-country Staffing and Administration	CDC/USAID	1,230,000	NA	Salary, travel and in-country support for resident advisors
Peace Corps third year volunteer	USAID	10,000	NA	Housing and travel for one volunteer
SUBTOTAL – In-country Staffing and Admin	CDC/USAID	**1,240,000**	**0**	
GRAND TOTAL		**24,000,000**	**12,920,500**	

www.ingramcontent.com/pod-product-compliance
Lightning Source LLC
Chambersburg PA
CBHW081244280526
45787CB00006B/2788